BRADY

Foundations for the Practice of EMS Education

Melissa Alexander, MS, NREMT-P
University of New Mexico EMS Academy

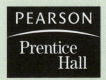

PEARSON
Prentice
Hall

Upper Saddle River, New Jersey 07458

Library of Congress Cataloging-in-Publication Data

Alexander, Melissa.
    Foundations for the practice of EMS education / Melissa Alexander.
        p. cm.
    Includes bibliographical references and index.
    ISBN 0-13-119435-6
    1. Emergency medical services—Study and teaching. 2. Emergency medical
personnel—Training of. I. Title.

RC645.5.A54 2006
616.02'5'0715—dc22

2005051500

Publisher: Julie Levin Alexander
Publisher's Assistant: Regina Bruno
Executive Editor: Marlene McHugh Pratt
Senior Acquisitions Editor: Stephen Smith
Senior Managing Editor
    for Development: Lois Berlowitz
Associate Editor: Monica Moosang
Editorial Assistant: Diane Edwards
Executive Marketing Manager: Katrin Beacom
Director of Marketing: Karen Allman
Marketing Coordinator: Michael Sirinides
Director of Production and
    Manufacturing: Bruce Johnson

Managing Production Editor: Patrick Walsh
Production Liaison: Julie Li
Production Editor: Karen Fortgang, bookworks
Manufacturing Manager: Ilene Sanford
Manufacturing Buyer: Pat Brown
Senior Design Coordinator: Cheryl Asherman
Interior Designer: Amy Rosen
Cover Designer: Michael Ginsberg
Cover Image: Jose Luis Pelaez, Inc./Corbis
Composition: The GTS Companies/York, PA Campus
Printing and Binding: R.R. Donnelley & Sons,
                                Harrisonburg
Cover Printer: Phoenix Color Corporation

Pearson Education LTD
Pearson Education Singapore, Pte. Ltd
Pearson Education Canada, Ltd
Pearson Education—Japan
Pearson Education Australia PTY, Limited

Pearson Education North Asia Ltd
Pearson Educación de Mexico, S.A. de C.V.
Pearson Education Malaysia, Pte. Ltd
Pearson Education, Upper Saddle River, New Jersey

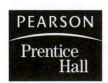

10 9 8 7 6 5 4 3 2 1
ISBN 0-13-119435-6

To Lindsay, Brittany, and Eleanor,
whose belief in me inspires me to persevere.

Contents

Chapter 5 Qualities, Competencies, Roles and Responsibilities of EMS Educators   53

Chapter 6 The Traits and Needs of Learners   75

Chapter 7 The Psychology of Learning   99

Chapter 8 Overview of the Educational Planning and Curriculum-Development Processes   117

Chapter 9 **Determining and Communicating Educational Needs   131**

Chapter 10 **Developing Instructional Objectives   151**

Chapter 11 **Packaging the Program   163**

Chapter 12 **Program Evaluation   177**

Chapter 13   Educational Measurement   189

Chapter 14   Student Evaluation and Remediation   207

Chapter 15   Selection of Materials and Media   237

Chapter **21**   **Career and Professional Development   309**

References   321

Answers   331

Index   352

Preface

This is a book about teaching, but even more so, it is about learning—both yours and your students'. Ultimately, all learning is personal. We create our knowledge through reflection on our experiences, constantly modifying or reinforcing the knowledge we already had based on earlier experiences. Just as importantly, all learning takes place in a context. Being an educator is not just something one does, but it is a way of thinking. I have endeavored to create a context of values and ideas through which to consider and apply the principles and practices of education. It is my hope that as you read this book, you will begin to think about your own thinking and learning and about how your own experiences, assumptions, and values shape your learning. In this way, you can animate the facts, theories, and principles in this book and bring them alive in your own practice as an educator.

This book cannot be an inexhaustible source of information on such a vast and complex field as education. It does provide sound, broad-based foundational knowledge with which to anchor further learning. I hope you will see it as a place to begin to learn (or to learn more) about education. As such, I have provided numerous resources for additional information for avenues you may wish to explore further. I also hope you will revisit this book from time to time after your initial reading and reconsider its contents in the context of your ongoing experiences as an educator.

This is an exciting time in EMS education, as we are poised to have tremendous impact on the future of EMS. Our first priority in realizing the potential of EMS is to develop a strong infrastructure of EMS educators, programs, and educational institutions. It has long been a dream of mine to put together in text form an organized collection of information and ideas to share with beginning educators and colleagues, alike. The skeleton of this text is the 2002 National Highway Traffic Safety Administration Guidelines for EMS Educators. I have fleshed out the skeleton with pieces on educational philosophy and theory, examples, and insights. Armed with content knowledge, educational process expertise, and shared values for education, we, as educators, will play a critical role in advancing both the EMS Agenda for the Future and the EMS Education Agenda for the Future.

Acknowledgments

There are many people without whose help, directly or indirectly, this book would not be possible. I am grateful for having three mentors, without whose support I would not have evolved in my career to the point where this undertaking was possible. I thank Peter Dillman, Steve Mercer, and Dan Limmer for their belief in me, encouragement, and provision of opportunities for professional development. I thank my original editor, Tiffany Price Salter, current editors Marlene Pratt and Stephen Smith, assistant editor Monica Moosang, and all those involved in copyediting and production of this book. I would also like to thank the reviewers of the original manuscript for their feedback and suggestions:

CHRISTOPHER BLACK
EMS Director
Eastern Arizona College
Thatcher, Arizona

KIM DICKERSON, EMT-P, RN
EMS Coordinator
Edison College
Fort Myers, Florida

STEPHEN L. GARRISON, RN, NREMT-P
EMS Manager
Memorial Hospital
South Bend, Illinois

JANE MACARTHUR, EMT-I/C
Executive Director
StarFire EMS
EMS Program Coordinator
Middlesex Community College
EMS Coordinator
Northern Essex Community College
Massachusetts

RICHARD W. SHOOK, EMT-B
Adjunct Faculty, SUNY Ulster
Department of Nursing and Public Safety Training
Stone Ridge, New York

BRIAN TURNER, BA, EMT-P
Northwestern Health Sciences University
Bloomington, MN

The Context
of EMS Education

Learning Objectives

Upon completion of this chapter you should be able to

- Appreciate the scope of adult education as a discipline.

- Discuss the relationship between adult education, higher education, and EMS education.

- Discuss significant documents that have shaped the course of EMS education.

- Present an overview of the entry-level competencies for EMS educators.

- Articulate the vision of the EMS Education Agenda for the Future.

CASE
Study_____

Prospective paramedic students Ben Larson and Trey Hartwell are considering application to several paramedic programs in their area. Nineteen-year-old Ben has been an EMT-Basic for nearly 2 years. He is single and lives at home with his parents and two sisters. His father has been a paramedic for 25 years. Ben would ultimately like to work his way into a position with a state or federal agency responsible for disaster planning. Trey, who just turned 25, has a bachelor's degree in agricultural science and plans to volunteer as a paramedic in his rural community. Ben and Trey have visited the Web sites for all of the programs but are still having some difficulties deciding which program would be best for each of them.

Questions

1. In what types of settings might Ben and Trey find a program to meet their individual career and personal needs?
2. How has EMS education changed since Ben's father became a paramedic?
3. What questions might Ben and Trey ask about the qualifications of their potential instructors?

Introduction

When approaching any field of study, it is useful to know the context in which it is situated and the events that shaped its evolution. This chapter gives an overview of the context of EMS education and discusses how adult education and higher education relate to EMS education. The foremost goal of this chapter, though, is to take you through the influential documents that have led us to the point where we are now in EMS education.

KEY TERMS

affective, p. 10

cognitive, p. 10

competency, p. 9

curricula, p. 6

curriculum, p. 5

enabling objective, p. 9

formative evaluation, p. 10

psychomotor, p. 11

summative evaluation, p. 10

terminal objective, p. 8

Adult Education and Adult Learning

Adult education is a broad field with a significant history as a specific discipline. Adult education activities range from English as a second language (ESL) courses offered by community organizations to fitness classes at the local gym, professional development courses through employers and professional associations, and a variety of other learning activities in which adults participate, either individually or in groups. Adult education as an endeavor differs in purpose from higher education, although this distinction is becoming less clear as more adults enter higher education programs. No matter the setting, principles of adult education and learning apply to EMS education.

The most difficult aspect of understanding adult education is figuring out what an adult is, because the criterion of chronological age is insufficient to explain what it is to be an adult. EMS National Standard Curricula are based on the assumption that the learners in our programs are adults, so although we will return to the topic of the adult learner in later chapters, this is an important point worthy of some consideration before we move on.

Considerations in Defining Adulthood

Adulthood is based upon many factors, including chronological age, sociocultural roles, and psychological maturity. It is important to recognize, though, that the mental processes by which people learn are not different between age groups. What differs between age groups is the amount and nature of experiences they have and the barriers to educational performance they may face. What makes an adult is the adaptation of thought and behavior based upon reflection on experiences, a process that takes place over time. This is the essence of maturity. The concept of experience is also important to the schools of philosophy of adult education discussed in the next chapter, as well as to models of adult learning presented later in the text.

Because EMS students are taking upon themselves the considerable responsibility that comes with being EMS providers, we must hold them accountable as adults. However, we deal with many young EMS students who may still be in high school or who have recently graduated from high school. Their life roles and responsibilities in most cases are not those that we would consider to be fully adult. They are a population in transition from adolescence to adulthood. The behavior and expectations of these students is often incongruent with what you will later learn about the nature of adult learners. It is important to realize that, although certainly not children, many of our students come to the classroom feeling entitled to be treated as adults. They do not yet have the experiences necessary to achieve adulthood, and this may be reflected in their conduct.

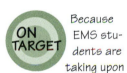

Because EMS students are taking upon themselves the considerable responsibility that comes with being EMS providers, we must hold them accountable as adults.

Although these behaviors are not necessarily restricted to the youngest students, often the lack of maturity manifests as holding others responsible for outcomes over which the student had control, but about which he or she made poor decisions. As an illustration, one of the more common situations occurs in scheduling clinical rotations. Younger students are frequently not able to prioritize clinical rotations in their social schedules and often at the end of the semester, when they realize that their clinical obligations are far from complete, the reason they give is that there weren't enough rotations scheduled. In contrast, students with adult roles and responsibilities outside the classroom usually come to the instructor early in the semester to discuss how they can work around other obligations that they must meet. Nonetheless, because of the responsibility shouldered by EMS providers, we can rightfully hold all students to expectations for adult behavior. Accordingly, this text approaches EMS education from the standpoint of adult education, with the caveat that not all students' behavior is consistent with societal expectations for adult conduct. As EMS educators, we sometimes need to guide students' experiences and their reflections on those experiences in a manner to help them grow and develop toward adulthood.

Definitions of Adult Education

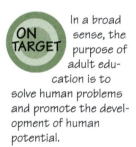

In a broad sense, the purpose of adult education is to solve human problems and promote the development of human potential.

Many definitions of adult education, including those of John Dewey and Eduard Lindeman, who are discussed in the next chapter, focus on the purpose of adult education as social reform and social action. It may be somewhat difficult to see how EMS education fits into such definitions of adult education. The foregoing definitions were conceived of in the early part of the twentieth century in a different sociopolitical climate than currently exists. It may make more sense in contemporary circumstances in first-world countries, such as the United States and Canada, to think of the broader purpose of adult education as being to solve human problems and promote the development of human potential. In this sense, it is much easier to see how EMS education fits into the definition of adult education.

Adult Education and Learning

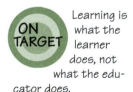

Learning is what the learner does, not what the educator does.

Adult education and adult learning are two distinct processes. Adult learning is an activity of the learner. It is what the learner does, not what the educator does. To illustrate, learning can take place in the context of a formal course or program and also takes place in an informal manner on a daily basis as the learner encounters various situations. Later in the text we spend more time considering the nature and needs of the adult learner. Adult education, on the other hand, takes place via planned, organized programs of study. To illustrate, consider Darkenwald and Merriam's definition of adult education: "Adult education is a process whereby persons whose major social roles are characteristic of adult status undertake systematic and sustained learning activities for the purpose of bringing about changes in knowledge, attitudes, values, or skills" (1982, 9).

Higher Education

EMS education is increasingly taking place in, or under the auspices of, institutions of higher education such as community colleges and universities, especially at levels above EMT-Basic. This is one of the goals of the EMS Agenda for the Future (NHTSA 1996) and has many benefits for the quality of EMS education. EMS programs conducted by accredited institutions of higher education are subject to curriculum oversight, program evaluation, and, in many cases, input from advisory committees. Institutions of higher learning can also offer considerable resources in terms of libraries, technology, and student services. This is not to imply that quality programs cannot be conducted in other settings, but other settings may have difficulty supporting the infrastructure to reinforce the program. Conversely, being anchored in an educational institution does not automatically lead to a quality EMS education program. This is where program accreditation, about which you will later learn more, plays a role.

There are benefits of higher-education affiliation to the EMS student, too. College credit is available for many EMT-Basic, EMT-Intermediate, and EMT-Paramedic programs, facilitating career and personal development. College-credit programs are also more likely to allow the student to qualify for financial aid. If your goal as an EMS educator is to teach in a higher-education setting, it is increasingly likely that you will be required to hold academic credentials at least one level above the credential granted by the program in which you are teaching. For example, if you will be teaching in a community college course that offers a certificate program, you most likely will need at least an associate's degree in a relevant area; and if you are teaching in an associate degree program, you will most likely need at least a bachelor's degree.

EMS Education

curriculum
A comprehensive plan to guide educational programming and processes.

The history of EMS education is linked to the evolution of EMS, overall. Although there were some elementary guidelines for physicians and nurses who trained ambulance attendants as early as the 1950s, the need for EMS educational standards was first recognized when the now historic 1966 report *Accidental Death and Disability: The Neglected Disease of Modern Society* was published by the National Academy of Sciences, National Research Council. The recognition that basic measures in the prehospital setting could significantly impact survival from automobile trauma led to federal funding for the development of EMS systems and the development of the first EMT-Ambulance standard **curriculum**, which was completed in 1971. The first national standard

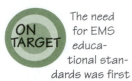

The need for EMS educational standards was first recognized when the now historic report *Accidental Death and Disability: The Neglected Disease of Modern Society* was published in 1966.

curricula
Plural of curriculum.

paramedic curriculum was developed in 1977. Although these efforts represent a colossal step forward for EMS, these **curricula** were developed largely in the absence of input from stakeholders in the profession and, as a result, the curricula have been a point of controversy in the field. Although some process changes were made in the revision and re-development of EMS curricula through the 1980s and 1990s, many stakeholders in the EMS community remained dissatisfied with both the methods and products of the processes.

The EMS Agenda for the Future

In 1996, the EMS Agenda for the Future (NHTSA) provided a vision for improved EMS education. The EMS Agenda for the Future, sponsored by NHTSA and the Health Resources and Services Administration (HRSA), Maternal and Child Health Bureau, outlines 14 aspects of EMS for ongoing development:

- Integration of health services
- EMS research
- Legislation and regulation
- System finance
- Human resources
- Medical direction
- Education systems
- Public education
- Prevention
- Public access
- Communications systems
- Clinical care
- Information systems
- Evaluation

It is easy to see that EMS educators have an important role to play in the development and execution of many of these elements. The document sets forth a vision (Box 1-1) and specific goals for EMS education. These goals significantly impact the required scope of educational process expertise that must be available to every EMS education program. Although it is not necessary for all EMS educators to achieve educational expertise beyond classroom teaching, it is necessary for all EMS educators to be familiar with the goals of the agenda. There are many activities based on these goals taking place at the national level. The documents and guidelines developed through these activities will

(*continued on page* 8)

Box 1-1

Vision of EMS Education from the EMS Agenda for the Future
(NHTSA 1996)

EMS education in the year 2010 develops competence in the areas necessary for EMS providers to serve the health-care needs of the population. Educational outcomes for EMS providers are congruent with the expectations of the health and public safety services that provide them. EMS education emphasizes the integration of EMS within the overall health-care system. In addition to acute emergency care, all EMS educational programs teach illness and injury prevention, risk modification, the treatment of chronic conditions, as well as community and public health.

EMS education is of high quality and represents the intersection of the EMS professional and the formal educational system. The content of the education is based on nationally developed National EMS Education Standards. There is significant flexibility to adapt to local needs and develop creative instructional programs. Programs are encouraged to excel beyond minimum educational quality standards. EMS education is based on sound educational principles and is broadly recognized as an achievement worthy of formal academic credit.

Basic level EMS education is available in a variety of traditional and non-traditional settings. Advanced level EMS education is sponsored by institutions of higher education and most are available for college credit. Multiple entry options exist for advanced level education, including bridging from other occupations, basic EMS levels and for individuals with no previous medical or EMS experience. All levels of EMS education are available through a variety of distance learning and creative, alternative delivery formats.

Educational quality is assured through a system of accreditation. This system evaluates programs relative to standards and guidelines developed by the national communities of interest. Entry level competence is assured by a combination of curricula standards, national accreditation, and national standard testing.

Licensure is based upon the completion of an approved/accredited program and successful completion of the national exam. This enables career mobility, advancement, and facilitates reciprocity and recognition for all levels.

Interdisciplinary and bridging programs provide avenues for EMS providers to enhance their credentials or transition to other health career roles, and for other health care professionals to acquire EMS field provider credentials. They facilitate adaptation of the work force as community health care needs, and the role of EMS, evolves.

impact the practice of every EMS educator. The goals for educational systems outlined in the EMS Agenda for the Future are as follows:

- Ensure adequacy of EMS education programs.
- Update educational core content objectives frequently enough so that they reflect patients' EMS health-care needs.
- Incorporate research, quality improvement, and management learning objectives in higher-level EMS education.
- Commission the development of national core contents to replace EMS program curricula.
- Conduct EMS education with medical direction.
- Seek accreditation for EMS education programs.
- Establish innovative and collaborative relationships between EMS education programs and academic institutions.
- Recognize EMS education as an academic achievement.
- Develop bridging and transition programs.
- Include EMS-related objectives in all health professions' education.

 PEARLS The EMS Agenda for the Future and the EMS Education Agenda for the Future are the leading documents in the development of the future of EMS and EMS Education.

The EMS Education Agenda for the Future

Because education is a core factor in the realization of progress in EMS, it has received special attention via the EMS Education Agenda for the Future, which expands upon the goals outlined in the EMS Agenda for the Future. The EMS Education Agenda for the Future (NHTSA 2000) puts forward five components for national EMS education, including Core Content, a Scope of Practice Model, Education Standards, Program Accreditation, and Certification. One of the major changes anticipated is that NHTSA will no longer sponsor the development of EMS curricula with detailed declarative information. Instead, through a series of processes laid out in the Education Agenda, a much less-directive set of educational standards, which will serve as **terminal objectives,** will be extracted from the national core content for each nationally recognized level of practice.

Whereas, to date, many EMS educators are using the detailed declarative information in the curricula as lesson plans (which is not the

terminal objective
A statement of an ultimate intended learning outcome. Also called *competency*.

intended application of such materials), EMS educators will be called upon to create **enabling objectives** and lesson plans from the educational standards. Many current EMS textbooks and instructor support materials are written directly from the declarative content of the National Standard Curricula. This practice will consequently change as well, requiring the EMS educator to develop skills in using textbooks as adjuncts, as they are intended to be, rather than using textbooks as course content.

National Guidelines for EMS Educators

The evolution of EMS education over the next several years will bring many changes and challenges to EMS educators. Although change is not easy, these changes are necessary to elevate EMS to the level it needs to be to meet the challenges facing it now and in the future. In recognition of the changes intended in EMS practice and EMS education, The National Association of EMS Educators (NAEMSE), in 2001 under agreement with the United States Department of Transportation (USDOT) National Highway Traffic Safety Administration (NHTSA), formed a task force to create new EMS instructor development guidelines. The goal of these guidelines, which serve as the core of this text, is to prepare entry-level EMS educators to meet a standard set of basic **competencies** in classroom instruction.

Professional Attributes and Skill Sets of EMS Instructors Defined by the EMS Instructor Development Task Force

The EMS Instructor Development Task Force defined 10 areas of competence for entry-level EMS educators, as follows:

- The EMS educator understands the central concepts, tools of inquiry, and structures of the EMS discipline(s) they teach and can create learning experiences that make these aspects of subject matter meaningful for the adult learner.
- The EMS educator understands how adult students learn and can provide learning opportunities that support their intellectual, professional, and personal development.
- The EMS educator understands how adult learners differ in their approaches to learning and creates instructional opportunities that can be adapted to diverse learning styles and situations.

formative evaluation
Assessment of the effectiveness of an educational program and/or student achievement while the program is on-going.

summative evaluation
Assessment of educational program effectiveness and/or student achievement at the end of an educational program.

cognitive
The domain of learning that pertains to the acquisition and processing of knowledge, to include application of the knowledge to new situations and solving problems not previously encountered.

affective
The domain of learning that pertains to the emotions, attitudes, and values associated with professional practice.

- The EMS educator understands and uses a variety of instructional strategies to encourage the adult learners' development of high-level thinking skills, problem-solving skills, and psychomotor performance skills.
- The EMS educator uses an understanding of individual and group motivation and behavior to create a learning environment that encourages positive group interaction, active engagement in learning, and self-motivation.
- The EMS educator uses knowledge of effective verbal, nonverbal, and media communication techniques to foster active inquiry, collaboration, and supportive interaction in the classroom.
- The EMS educator plans instruction based upon knowledge of subject matter, the attributes of the adult learner, and curriculum goals.
- The EMS educator understands and uses **formative** and **summative evaluation** strategies with both formal and informal techniques to evaluate and ensure the continuous **cognitive, affective,** and **psychomotor** development of the learner.
- The EMS educator is a reflective practitioner who continually evaluates the effects of [his or her] choices and actions on others (the adult learner and other professionals in the learning community) and who actively seeks out opportunities to grow professionally.
- The EMS educator fosters relationships with EMS colleagues and EMS agencies in the larger community to support the students' learning and well-being.
(NHTSA 2002)

We return to these competencies in greater detail throughout the remainder of the text, because it is the goal of this text to assist you in developing the skills and knowledge necessary to demonstrate the attributes of an entry level EMS educator.

Summary

EMS education sits in the overlapping contexts of adult education and higher education. This makes a brief overview of adult education and learning and the influence of higher education on EMS education relevant to the EMS educator. EMS education has found its way into these contexts from its beginnings as elementary guidelines for the training of ambulance attendants by physicians and nurses in the 1950s. Because of the demands for EMS to progress to a higher level of service to the community, EMS education is evolving into a complex endeavor that recognizes the importance of sound educational processes for developing core

psychomotor
The domain of learning that pertains to the skilled performance of tasks requiring physical dexterity.

content and educational standards. The core content and educational standards must be operationalized by individuals who are not just expert practitioners, but who are proficient in educational processes as well. NAEMSE, under contract with NHTSA and in response to the vision set forth by the EMS Agenda for the Future, has developed standards for the minimum competencies required of the entry-level classroom teacher. The goal of this text is to serve as a resource and guide for developing these competencies.

REVIEW QUESTIONS

1. What document heralded the beginning of EMS education as we know it today?

2. What two documents are currently shaping the future of EMS and EMS education?

3. What organization has developed national guidelines for EMS educators?

4. What is the primary difference between adult learners and younger learners?

5. List five competencies required of EMS educators.

Philosophical Foundations of Education

Learning Objectives

Upon completion of this chapter you should be able to

- Describe the value of studying educational philosophy.

- Describe the basic frameworks of progressive education and humanistic education.

- Give examples of learning activities consistent with the principles of progressive education and humanistic education.

- Explain how elements of progressivism and humanism can be incorporated into competency-based National Standard EMS curricula.

CASE Study____

Rita Bowes has just finished teaching her first "solo" EMT-Intermediate class. She has just received her course evaluations and is talking about them to her colleague Anne Barnes, an experienced EMS educator. "The students were really hard on me for not posting copies of my lecture notes and PowerPoint® presentations online," Rita says. "I don't believe the students learn as well from that as they would by paying attention to the case studies and discussions in class and asking questions. On the other hand," she continues, "I don't want to get poor teaching evaluations. What should I do?"

Questions

1. Although the students are most likely unaware of different philosophies of education, from what philosophical perspective do you think they are coming?
2. How is the students' philosophical perspective different than Rita's?
3. If you were Anne, what advice would you give to Rita?

Introduction

You may be wondering why it is necessary, for the purposes of EMS education, to consider philosophy. This can be best answered by the following often-used quote (original source unknown): "Philosophy without practice is useless, and practice without philosophy is blind." So, as you can see, the purpose of a philosophy of education is to guide our actions and practices as educators. As John Dewey said, "The need for a philosophy of education is fundamentally the need for finding out what education really is" (Archambault 1964, 4). There are two standpoints from which philosophy of education can be addressed. First, educational philosophy is a formal field of study based in broader philosophical roots. There are several schools of philosophical thought that inform educational practice. Two of these schools are particularly relevant to the context of EMS education: progressive education and humanistic education. In this chapter we explore how each of these philosophies views the nature of human beings, what constitutes knowledge, and educational practices that are consistent with these philosophies. We also touch briefly on the liberal and behavioral philosophies of education by way of comparison.

schemata
Plural of schema.

schema
An individual's mental script for things or events.

The second way in which educational philosophy can be viewed is as a set of personal beliefs and values related to the practice of education. In this informal manner, we all have philosophies regarding a wide variety of social interactions. Although we seldom consciously examine our personal philosophies, we create what we call **schemata** based on our personal philosophies and prior experiences with objects and events. A **schema** is a mental roadmap or script for the way we believe particular situations should play out or for how people should be or act in particular situations.

Using Formal and Personal Philosophies

Chris Argyris (1982) writes that we have both an *espoused theory*, and a *theory-in-use* for the things that we do. Usually, there is a gap between what we say we believe, the espoused theory, and what we actually do, our theory-in-use. Gaining a better understanding of formal educational philosophies can help us think about the assumptions of our own philosophies, help us to build and refine our personal philosophies, and help us modify our practices so that our espoused theories and theories-in-use become more consistent with each other. Like educators, learners also have personal philosophies of education and, thus, schemata that guide their beliefs about learning and the roles of the learner and teacher (Tisdell and Taylor 2000). It is not uncommon for there to be conflict between students' and teachers' beliefs about the teaching-learning transaction. Having a basic understanding of formal educational philosophy and the educational approaches consistent with them will help you feel surer of your practices and decisions when they are challenged by students, as they are apt to be.

 PEARLS It is good practice to ask yourself whether your planned methods of instruction are consistent with your beliefs about learning.

Philosophy versus Theory

Before we proceed with the details of the two philosophies under consideration in this chapter, it is important to distinguish between *philosophy* and *theory*, because the line between them is often blurred. In fact, some authors (Merriam and Caffarella 1999) have chosen to describe general orientations toward learning that each encompasses a number of theories with similar philosophical bases (Table 2-1).

Table 2-1

Orientation to Learning	Major Theorists	Purpose of Education	Role of the Educator	Implications for Learning	Application in EMS Education
Behaviorist	Pavlov, Skinner, Watson, Thorndike	Produce a desired change in behavior	Arranges the environment to produce a response	Behavioral objectives, competency-based education, skills training	Curriculum development, lesson-planning, testing, and evaluation
Cognitivist	Gagne, Piaget	Develop capacity and skills for learning	Structures content of learning activity	Learning how to learn, intelligence, memory	Learning strategies, student remediation
Humanist	Maslow, Rogers	Self-actualization, autonomy	Facilitates development of whole person	Self-directed learning	Teacher-learner relationship, motivation, continuing education
Social Learning	Bandura	Model new roles and behavior	Models roles and behaviors, guides learner in adoption of roles and behaviors	Mentoring	Clinical education, new employee orientation
Constructivist	Dewey, Kolb	Construction of knowledge from experience	Assists learner in finding meaning in experience	Experiential learning, reflective practice	Teaching strategies, laboratory education, clinical education, continuing education

Adapted from Merriam, S. B., and R. S. Caffarella, 1999. *Learning in adulthood: A comprehensive guide,* 2d ed. San Francisco: Jossey-Bass.

Philosophy

A **philosophy** is a broad system of values and beliefs regarding the nature of things, based on logical reasoning rather than on observation or experience. The purpose of philosophy is to make sense of the world, to find the meaning of things. As noted before, at the core of a philosophy are some very basic issues regarding the nature of the world, the nature of human beings, and the nature of "knowing." Every person has a set of values and beliefs; a philosophy that guides his or her behavior. A philosophy of education guides the educator in his or her practice of education, whether he or she has examined that philosophy or not. Part of the value of studying philosophies of education is to find a philosophy that resonates with one's own belief system. This helps educators to think more deeply about the nature of the human beings with whom they will be working and to use approaches to education that are consistent with those beliefs.

Theory

A **theory** is a limited set of assumptions and the principles derived from those assumptions, which help to predict, explain, or analyze a specific phenomenon, such as how people learn. Theories can be derived from observations in qualitative research and, once developed, can be used to guide further qualitative and quantitative research. Theories often have models associated with them to help illustrate how a phenomenon occurs. Theories certainly have their bases in philosophy, but address a very specific type of occurrence, rather than the general nature of the world.

Philosophies of Education

A philosophy is a broad way of viewing things, whereas a theory offers an explanation of how or why something occurs.

Progressive Education

Progressive versus Liberal Education

The foundation of the progressive philosophy of education is pragmatism, a larger philosophy of the nature of meaning in the world. Pragmatism focuses on those things that are useful or practical. This is in contrast to **liberal education,** which has an intellectual focus that emphasizes the acquisition of a body of knowledge laden with philosophy, humanities, and religion. Liberal education has its beginnings in ancient Greece and was developed in the context of the elite of a society in which work was performed by an underclass. Science and work-related

liberal education
A classic approach to education that focuses on the subject matter of the humanities and deemphasizes science.

progressive education
An approach to knowledge based on observation, experimentation, and applicability.

content are deemphasized in liberal education. Liberal education is based on a relatively static body of knowledge and is authoritarian in nature. The teacher is viewed as an expert, whose job it is to impart knowledge. The student is more or less a passive container, whose role it is to absorb and store the knowledge imparted. It is important to note that much of what occurs in the American public school system is based in the liberal tradition and that this has shaped the expectations of the students in your classroom.

Progressive education has a more scientific approach to knowledge, an approach based in observation, experimentation, and applicability. Progressivism, although conceived of by John Dewey as an approach to education in the American school system, has had an enormous influence on adult education. Many of the renowned theorists in the field of adult education, including Malcolm Knowles, Cyril Houle, Eduard Lindeman, David Kolb, and others, have adopted the progressive approach originated by John Dewey. The purpose of progressive education is to learn what is useful in life (Dewey 1938). More important and useful than any particular subject matter or skill is the ability to think rationally and reflectively on experiences in order to solve new problems. This is manifest in the 1998 Paramedic NSC (NHTSA 1998), in which clinical problem solving and critical thinking are explicitly addressed.

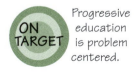

Progressivism is concerned with learning to think rationally and reflectively on experiences in order to solve new problems.

The Progressive Approach to Learning and Teaching

The progressive view of human beings is that they are naturally inclined toward rationality and seek the truth through experimentation. Learning is an active process undertaken by the learner. He or she is not a passive store of facts, but rather creates knowledge through reflection on experiences. One of the roles of the educator is to guide the learner in developing powers of reflection and reconstruction of experience. By reconstruction of experience we mean that reflection on a new experience modifies or refines what we have learned from previous experience, thus reconstructing it. This process of reconstruction occurs continually, so that there is not an end to learning. Progressive education is problem centered. For example, a progressive educational approach would be to pose a problem, such as a case study, at the beginning of class. It is then for the purpose of solving this problem that subject matter becomes relevant to the learner. Another essential role of the progressive educator is that of a guide who, on the basis of his or her greater experience, directs education toward experiences that meet the learners' needs. This means that, as educators, we must have an idea of how our students' prior experiences fit with the subject matter at hand. As you will see in later chapters, students' prior experiences can both facilitate and hinder new learning.

ON TARGET Progressive education is problem centered.

The Nature of Experience

Experience, as you've noted, is a central concept in progressivism. As such, it is worthwhile to briefly consider what constitutes an experience. An experience occurs as a result of interaction between an individual and his or her environment. The progressive educator has a role in creating an authentic environment with which the student can interact. The richer the environment is in stimuli that emulate the real world, the more reflective the learning will be of what is expected in the real world. Methods of progressive education are those in which the learner is an active participant and include strategies such as observation, case studies, role-playing, simulation, and guided real-life experiences. The progressive educator then asks a series of questions to provoke reflection on the experience. We know that learning has occurred when the student can then apply that experience to a new experience in order to solve a problem he or she has not previously encountered.

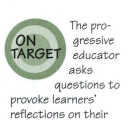

The progressive educator asks questions to provoke learners' reflections on their experiences.

Not all experiences are of equal educational value. The value of an experience is determined by its continuity with other experiences, promotion of growth in a positive direction, and advancement of positive mental habits and approaches to further learning. According to Dewey (1938), experiences that do not meet these criteria are *miseducative*. The concept of continuity is demonstrated by the certainty that every experience is affected by those that came before it and affects those that occur after it. This is a critical concept to which we return in later chapters. The development of positive mental habits is a process of recognizing the relationships between ideas and the ability to apply them in new situations. The progressive educator is concerned with arranging experiences in a manner that promotes reflection and calls upon the student to apply the ideas distilled from that reflection to solving new problems. In fact, it has been said that the unexamined experience is not worth having.

The Role of Subject Matter in Experiential Learning

This explanation of progressivism is not meant to imply that traditional subject matter has no place in education. Whereas in liberal education, taking in the subject matter itself is the goal of learning, progressivists view subject matter as a source of experience that can be used in solving problems. The progressive educator must take care to situate subject matter in a curriculum in a manner that takes into account the learner's experiences and needs. What we have learned through progressivism is that subject matter must be arranged logically, in a sequence beginning with what the learner already knows, progressing in a continuous fashion to what the learner needs to know.

Growth, or learning, occurs via the problem-solving method, in which we begin by clarifying the problem to be solved. We then develop ideas or hypotheses about the problem and test them on the basis of what we can observe. Case studies, simulation, and other methods of education with which you are no doubt familiar from your own EMS educational experience, were mentioned earlier. Whether you have realized it or not, you have used this approach in your own formal classroom learning in EMS, as well as in your experiences as a clinician when you approach patients. As an educator, you can enhance your students' learning by providing a framework for reflection on experiences and asking thought-provoking questions. One very effective way of doing this, about which you will learn more in later chapters, is to have students complete a short directed-journaling exercise in conjunction with each clinical rotation. As a developing educator, you will also find it helpful to include at the end of your lesson plans a few reflective questions directed to yourself, to be answered after you have completed the lesson.

Humanistic Education

Humanism Complements Progressivism

humanistic education
An approach to education that emphasizes the inherent dignity of human beings and their needs for meaning and growth.

It often happens that philosophers are at odds with each over the convictions of their particular philosophies, focusing on incongruencies rather than on complementary facets of the philosophies. In this particular case, humanistic educational philosophy can be quite complementary to progressivism. **Humanistic education** focuses on the needs and inherent dignity of human beings as its core. Humanism is concerned with the development of the whole person, including his or her emotional, psychological, social, and *affective* development. Humanistic influence can be seen in the current versions of EMS national standard curricula in the affective objectives stated in many of the lessons. Abraham Maslow's hierarchy of needs is a commonly recognized concept in humanistic philosophy. In terms of adult education, **andragogy** (a theory of adult learning), a term popularized by Malcolm Knowles, is based heavily on humanistic philosophy. We return to both Maslow and Knowles in later chapters as we discuss learning and motivation.

andragogy
A theory of education based on the needs and expectations of the adult learner.

ON TARGET A humanistic approach to education is based on a good relationship between the educator and the learners.

The Humanistic Approach to Learning and Teaching

The humanist view of humanity is that life is not inherently meaningful, but that each person must develop meaning in his or her life. Humanism is concerned with the full development of human potential. In this endeavor, a good relationship between teacher and student is essential to learning, although learning itself is intensely personal.

Some of the key concepts of humanism as they are applicable to a content-specific discipline such as EMS are as follows:

- A humanistic approach includes both *cognitive* and *affective* involvement of the learner.
- Motivation is intrinsic—it comes from within the learner.
- Learning is experiential.
- Learning is cooperative, not competitive.
- Individuals' uniqueness and experiences must be recognized and respected.
- There should be a focus on concern for the welfare of humankind.

Humanism in Perspective

The primary criticism of humanism is that it is too unstructured. This criticism should be viewed relative to the purpose of the educational endeavor. Humanism assumes that adult education is voluntary and is undertaken by an individual to meet a particular need. Because of the specific outcomes required of EMS education programs and because there are many situations in which students in EMS classrooms are not there completely of their own free will, a humanistic approach cannot be adopted as a whole for our purposes. However, many of the tenets of humanism are quite applicable both in the classroom and in clinical practice.

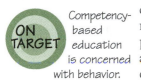

ON TARGET Competency-based education is concerned with behavior.

competency-based education
An approach to education based on learners' achievement of prespecified tasks of the occupation.

behavioral education
A theory of education concerned only with behavior change based on stimulus and response and not with the cognitive or affective domains of learning.

Behaviorism

To put this discussion on philosophy in context, note that the EMS National Standard Curricula that we are currently using are competency based. **Competency-based education** (CBE) is consistent with **behavioral education**, which takes a much different view of learning and human beings. The behaviorist focus is on changing human behavior through manipulation of the environment, such as by providing stimuli and consequences for behavior. Prominent behaviorists with whom you may be familiar include B. F. Skinner, E. L. Thorndike, and Ivan Pavlov. Behaviorists don't deny that there are human qualities such as insight, reasoning, feelings, and judgment; but since these qualities cannot be directly observed, they are not behaviorists' concern. It is important to remember that because we are in a discipline in which our competence to perform has enormous impact and is rightfully scrutinized, it is necessary to set forth minimum, entry-level standards, or competencies. However, within these curricula, there is plenty of room for the individual educator's philosophical approach to education to be exercised through the methods and activities he or she chooses as a means for assisting students in achieving the stated competencies.

Summary

Philosophy is a subject often approached with trepidation (or avoided altogether!) because of its complex and nebulous nature. Nonetheless, educational philosophy is useful as a guide to practice. Realizing that there are different philosophical approaches to education will also help you understand other educators' approaches and points of view. Recognition that each person, consciously or unconsciously, develops his or her own personal philosophy and schemata will help you understand the expectations that accompany learners into the classroom. You may have discovered through the discussion on espoused theories and theories-in-use that some of your own behaviors are inconsistent with philosophical tenets that ring true with you. This awareness can assist you in making your classroom actions and decisions consistent with your values. The goal of this chapter has been to acquaint you with two philosophies of education upon which theories discussed in later chapters are based. Completing the Philosophy of Adult Education Inventory©, developed by Lorraine Zinn, will help you identify the philosophy most similar to your beliefs. You can self-administer this inventory online by going to **http://www25.brinkster.com/educ605/paei_howtouse.htm** or **http://www.cals.ncsu.edu/agexed/aee523/paei.pdf**. You may then wish to read further about that philosophy and to compare and contrast it to other philosophies.

REVIEW QUESTIONS

1. Which philosophical perspective on education is most concerned with the dignity of human beings and their needs for growth?

2. What general orientation to learning is related to progressive philosophy?

3. Which philosophy of education serves as the basis for competency-based education?

Ethics, Standards, and Legal Considerations in EMS Education

Learning Objectives

Upon completion of this chapter you should be able to

- List sources of information regarding national, state, and local regulations, policies, and procedures related to EMS education programs.

- Defend the need for national, state, and local guidelines for EMS education programs.

- Discuss applicable federal, state, and local laws that affect the EMS teaching profession and the educational institution.

- Explain legal considerations regarding copyright and intellectual property issues.

- Define liability, negligence, and the standard of instruction.

- Identify areas of legal liability and risk-management considerations for the student, instructor, and educational institution.

- Explain the importance of confidentiality of student information.

- Differentiate between ethics and morals.

- Compare and contrast theories of morality as they relate to human development and conduct.

- Discuss the ethical position statement of NAEMSE and the NEA Code of Ethics.

- Provide examples of ethical and unethical instructor conduct.

- Describe the importance of ethical role models in the classroom, lab, and clinical settings of EMS education.

- Describe ways in which ethics can be incorporated into course curricula.

- Defend the need for instructors to adhere to principles of ethical and legal conduct in the practice of EMS education.

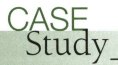

CASE Study

Neil Vance, a senior instructor in an EMS program, is waiting in his office to meet with the program director, Michelle Wong, regarding a student grievance. Two weeks ago one of Neil's students, Jim, whose academic performance was borderline throughout the semester, failed the dynamic cardiology station of the course's practical exam. The practical exam evaluator notified Neil and, according to course policy, the course medical director retested Jim with Neil present. Jim made several critical errors during the retest. According to program policy, Jim could not graduate from the program until retaking and passing EMP 221, the senior skills laboratory course.

Neil had talked to Jim about this at the time, and Jim admitted that he wasn't prepared and that he "really messed up." Neil talked to Jim about the next time the course would be offered and what Jim would need to do to register for it. Jim seemed accepting of this, so Neil was surprised when Michelle told him the reason for the meeting. During their meeting, Michelle told Neil that Jim was threatening to sue the institution if he was not allowed another retest because he felt that Neil did not like him and had been unfair to him all semester. Jim claimed that Neil had intimidated him by telling Jim that the treatment he proposed in a lab scenario many months before would be fatal to the patient.

Questions

1. Does it seem that Jim has a legitimate basis for requesting another retest?

2. What factors should be taken into consideration in deciding whether Jim should be allowed a retest?
3. Is it likely that Jim could sue the institution on the basis of his complaint of "intimidation" if denied a retest?
4. What ethical elements can you identify in this case?

Introduction

The purpose of this chapter is to discuss the administrative regulation of EMS education, areas of potential liability in the practice of EMS education, and the moral and ethical obligations of EMS education practitioners. Without knowledge of the particulars of these content areas, EMS educators could unwittingly find themselves facing student complaints, disciplinary action, and perhaps civil and/or criminal legal action. The actions of an EMS educator can affect the EMS education program, the larger institution housing the program, and the profession of EMS education. Therefore, it is important that you consider this information prior to learning the tasks and roles of the EMS educator. This way, as you acquire the knowledge and skills of an educator, you will be doing so in consideration of the legal and ethical context in which you must apply the knowledge and skills.

KEY TERMS

discrimination, p. 30	liability, p. 28	morals, p. 36
ethics, p. 36	litigation, p. 28	plagiarism, p. 33
harassment, p. 29	malpractice, p. 29	values, p. 36
indemnification, p. 36		

Sources of Information on Legal and Administrative Issues

The policies, procedures, and regulations of many different entities can affect the way an EMS program is conducted. These entities may be at the national, state, local, and/or institutional levels, depending upon the context and nature of your program. Regulations may apply to such issues as the length, format, content, and standards of educational programs,

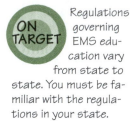

Regulations governing EMS education vary from state to state. You must be familiar with the regulations in your state.

instructor qualifications, student prerequisites for admission, student rights, certification and testing requirements, civil rights, equipment safety, and other areas. In addition to regulations and guidelines, many agencies and associations also offer resources such as educational materials, networking opportunities, continuing professional development opportunities, and grant funding. Therefore, you are encouraged to visit the websites of the agencies and associations listed in Boxes 3-1, 3-2, and 3-3. You can also go to the website **www.findlaw.com** to find information specific to your state.

Box 3-1

National Agencies and Associations

United States Department of Transportation/National Highway Traffic Safety Administration: **www.nhtsa.dot.gov/people/injury/ems**

Health Resources and Services Administration/Maternal Child Health Bureau/ EMS for Children: **http://www.mchb.hrsa.gov**

National Association of State EMS Directors: **www.nasemsd.org**

National Council of State EMS Training Coordinators: **www.ncsemstc.org**

American College of Emergency Physicians: **www.acep.org**

National Association of EMS Physicians: **www.naemsp.org**

National Registry of Emergency Medical Technicians: **www.NREMT.org**

Committee on Accreditation of Educational Programs for EMS Professionals: **www.coaemsp.org**

Continuing Education Coordinating Board for EMS: **www.cecbems.org**

American Society for Training and Development: **www.astd.org**

Federal Emergency Management Agency: **www.fema.gov**

National Association of EMTs: **www.NAEMT.org**

International Association of Fire Fighters: **www.iaff.org**

International Association of Fire Chiefs: **www.iafc.org**

National Association of EMS Educators: **www.NAEMSE.org**

Occupational Safety and Health Administration: **www.osha.gov**

Box3-2

State-Level Resources for EMS Educators

State EMS office or agency (may be part of a larger office, such as the state health department)

Google, searched using your state's name and "EMS" or "Office of EMS" (For example, the official website for the Virginia Office of EMS is easily found by searching for "Virginia Office of EMS.")

State EMS associations

State chapters of NAEMT

State EMS education associations

State laws and administrative codes

State's laws at **www.findlaw.com**

State divisions of federal offices such as OSHA

State commission on higher education

Program-Specific Considerations

Other specific sources of information regarding your program are important, too. Some resources that you should have immediately available to you include

- Faculty code and/or handbook.
- Employee handbook.

Box3-3

Local and Institutional Resources for EMS Educators

Local or regional EMS councils

College and University policies (often found on the institution's website)

Policies of other institutions for whom you may conduct programs (hospitals, fire departments, law-enforcement agencies, private companies, etc.)

- Your job description.
- Student handbook.
- Program policies.
- Course policies.
- Course syllabus.
- Contact information for the program administrator and/or medical director.

In some cases you will play a role in developing a program handbook, course policies, and/or syllabi. Some institutions may have guidelines for the development of these documents, whereas others see this as a discretionary task for the instructor or program administrator. Certain information is traditionally included in course policies, either as a separate document or included in the course syllabus. Any specific administrative information for which you want to hold students accountable must be included in the course or program policies. Often, course and program policies are a work in progress, with revisions made following occurrences that were not addressed by existing policy. If your institution does not provide a template or guideline, you may want to refer to the sample course syllabus in this text as a guide. Experienced instructors affiliated with your program or other programs in your area are also a good source of information regarding policies and practices that have worked for them.

Legal Considerations in EMS Education

liability
Legal responsibility.

litigation
Legal proceedings.

As an EMS educator you must be aware of actions or omissions that can lead to criminal prosecution and/or civil **liability** for you and/or your educational institution. Instructors and educational institutions are not immune from lawsuits, either warranted or unwarranted. Criminal prosecution can result from actions such as assault, battery, harassment, and discrimination. Civil **litigation** may arise for a variety of reasons either in conjunction with criminal prosecution or in the absence of criminal offense.

Although the classroom may seem relatively safe legally when compared to fieldwork, we live in a society where many people operate on a sense of entitlement rather than merit. It is not uncommon for students to feel entitled to pass a program because they have paid for it, even when they have failed to meet minimum competencies for reasons related to their own abilities or efforts. At times these students' efforts to get what they feel they are entitled to reach the level of threatened litigation. On the other hand, there are some instructors who fail to meet

malpractice
An act of improper practice of one's profession.

their obligations to students and who can be considered to have committed educational **malpractice.** Because of the litigation-oriented society in which we live, it is critical that EMS educators are aware of potential areas of liability and have clearly stated course policies for which students must sign to acknowledge receipt.

The Standard of Instruction

As a clinician you are no doubt familiar with the standard of care as it applies to EMS providers. A similar concept, standard of instruction, exists for educators. Like the standard of care, the standard of instruction represents the actions of a reasonable person with similar experience and education. Standards of care can be derived from textbooks, curricula, protocols, laws, and expert opinion. Although there is not a universally agreed-upon set of descriptions for standards of instruction, the EMS instructor curriculum, textbooks, instructor certification requirements, experts, and in some cases, laws can serve as the standard against which your actions can be judged.

Areas of Potential Liability for the EMS Educator

Some of the specific areas of potential liability for EMS educators include harassment, discrimination, student injury, patient injury, violation of provisions of the Americans with Disabilities Act (ADA), violation of provisions of the Family Educational Rights and Privacy Act (FERPA), and violation of the provisions of the Health Insurance Portability and Accountability Act (HIPAA).

Harassment

harassment
A series of acts of persecution meant to trouble or disturb another person.

Harassment is a series of acts of persecution meant to trouble or disturb another person. This can include a succession of annoyances, threats, and/or demands on another person. Although we often think of sexual harassment when we think of harassment, harassment can obviously take other forms. Many agencies and institutions offer educational programs on avoiding claims of sexual harassment or detecting sexual harassment when an employee or student is harassing a coworker or classmate. It is important to remember that, in civil litigation, it is necessary that a jury believe only that it is more likely that one person is telling the truth than the other. It is also important to remember that there is a difference between what one person's intent is and what another person's perception of the same behavior is. Nonetheless, there are some guidelines you should keep in mind to minimize claims of harassment:

- Use consistent and fair practices in dealing with all your students.
- Avoid situations in which you are alone with students (keep your office door open).
- Allow other instructors to evaluate the student's performance.
- Avoid intimate contact with students.
- Be aware of cultural differences in the expectation for personal space.
- Avoid suggestive statements or allowing students to make suggestive statements, because they may easily be misinterpreted.
- Make expectations for student conduct clear in policies.
- Have policies regarding revealing or suggestive dress, including T-shirts with slogans that may be offensive.

Discrimination

discrimination
Taking disparate action on the basis of prejudice; for example, unequal treatment based on gender, race, ethnicity, religion, sexual preference, or other differences.

Discrimination involves taking disparate action on the basis of prejudice—for example, unequal treatment based on gender, race, ethnicity, religion, sexual preference, or other differences. As with minimizing the chances of being accused of harassment, you must use consistent and fair policies in dealing with all students to minimize chances of being accused of discrimination. In addition, you should clearly document students' performance on practical evaluations and in clinical settings and use care to make grading decisions based on objective criteria. Of course, you should always analyze your own decisions for objectivity, and in cases where you feel it is possible that a student may claim discrimination, it is best to have multiple instructors (who may include your medical director and program director) evaluate the student's performance.

 PEARLS For evaluations that involve any subjectivity, it is important to have more than one instructor evaluate the student.

Student Injury

Litigation related to student injury can arise any time a student receives an injury while involved in the educational activities of your program. Injuries occurring in the clinical setting that can be attributed to instruction or program administration may be injuries related to improper instruction in the performance of a procedure, improper or inadequate supervision by a preceptor, or inadequate or malfunctioning equipment. Liability for student injury in the clinical setting must always be addressed in the clinical affiliation agreement or memorandum of understanding between a clinical agency and the educational program. It is essential that student competence in performing procedures be observed and documented in the laboratory setting prior to authorizing a student to perform those procedures in the clinical setting. Program policy must be clear about the circumstances under which students may perform procedures in the clinical setting.

Students can be injured in laboratory practice of skills, as well. Students must receive proper instruction before attempting a skill that may result in injury and must be supervised in skill practice. Again, course policy must be clear about student behavior in labs. Students should not be allowed to use equipment in a manner for which it was not intended, and extreme care must be taken when allowing students to practice skills on each other. Not only is there risk when students are practicing invasive skills such as injections and intravenous lines, but also when they are lifting, splinting, and practicing basic life-support skills. It is common for EMS education programs to receive used equipment that has been "retired" from service. It is essential that this equipment be examined carefully and that all lab equipment be regularly inspected and maintained. Many programs, because of the risks inherent in clinical and laboratory instruction, ask students to sign a waiver of liability for injury and/or an acknowledgment of the risks involved.

Patient Injury

Another source of potential liability for the EMS educator and/or the educational institution is injury to patients occurring from student actions. Once again, proper documentation of student skill performance in the laboratory, including drug-dosage calculation as well as the physical steps in skill performance, is an important step in avoiding liability. Course policy must be clear about what students can do and under what circumstances tasks can be performed. Clinical affiliation agreements or memoranda of understanding must address liability for student errors in the clinical setting. Preceptor education should emphasize proper supervision of students in the performance of patient interventions.

An additional consideration for protecting yourself and your institution against claims for student and patient injury is keeping instructional records, such as course syllabi, lesson plans, attendance records, exams, student test scores, and student skill-evaluation sheets. The purpose of such documentation is to provide evidence of what was taught in the class and how the student performed in class. This will prove valuable if a student claims that a particular skill or the knowledge associated with it was not taught. These items also provide a basis for evaluation of the quality of your program and are necessary for accreditation purposes. In most cases there are state and institutional guidelines concerning how long such records must be kept.

Americans with Disabilities Act (ADA)

The ADA requires that reasonable accommodations be made for individuals with documented disabilities. Although this seems like a fairly straightforward statement, there are two important points to consider here. The first is that the student's disability must be documented and he or she must make the educational institution aware of the disability. In other words, a student with dyslexia cannot, after failing an examination, for example, claim a violation of ADA if he or she did not previously make the instructor aware of the disability and provide appropriate documentation of the disability.

The second point is that the accommodations needed must be reasonable. A reasonable accommodation is one that could also be made to the person on the job as an EMS provider without interfering with the essential requirements of the job. For example, a paramedic student with a learning disability who requires longer to take written examinations would be likely to receive accommodations because reading speed is not addressed in the functional job analysis for the EMT-Paramedic (NHTSA 1999). In contrast, a student who is hearing impaired and needs a sign-language interpreter in class would most likely not be granted accommodations, because the functional job analysis requires that the paramedic be able to hear environmental stimuli. A situation that commonly arises is the student who requests that written examinations be read aloud. This accommodation is usually not granted, because the ability to read is a bona fide job requirement for which accommodations cannot be made on the job.

It is best that students requesting accommodations be referred to the appropriate student services or human resources personnel. Individuals in these positions are knowledgeable regarding ADA. Usually, student services can let the instructor know what type of accommodation is permitted. Your state EMS office can also provide you with information about accommodations permitted. The ADA can be found on the U.S. Department of Justice website at **www.usdoj.gov/crt/ada**.

Family Educational Rights and Privacy Act

The U.S. Congress enacted the Family Educational Rights and Privacy Act (FERPA), also known as the Buckley Amendment, in 1974 and made further amendments to it to strengthen the protection of privacy and other rights in 1994. FERPA applies to any educational agency that receives federal education funds. Under FERPA, educational records are considered to be all records that educational institutions or programs maintain about students. In postsecondary education, the student has the right to access and verify the accuracy of educational records. Students' rights to privacy are protected by regulations that restrict the release of information about students to certain legally defined instances. FERPA issues may arise when an employer who is paying for a particular student's education requests information about the student's performance in the program. Institutional and state regulations exist to support FERPA, and you must know the policies of your institution about the release of information. An additional issue is the posting of grades. When posting grades, no information that can be linked to an individual student, such as a student identification or social security number, may be used. FERPA is covered under Title 20 of the U.S. Code. Detailed information on FERPA can be found at **www.access.gpo.gov/uscode**, at **http://nces.ed.gov/pubs97/97859.html**, and through the U.S. Department of Education at **www.ed.gov/**.

Health Insurance Portability and Accountability Act

As an EMS professional you are no doubt familiar with the Health Insurance Portability and Accountability Act of 1996, which restricts the release and usage of patient information. It is also essential that your students be familiar with HIPAA prior to entering the clinical setting. In many cases the facilities and agencies with which your program has clinical affiliation agreements will insist on language in the contract to address student HIPAA training. Some of the instances that you should anticipate, and therefore address specifically with your students, include discussions about patients and copying patient information, lab results, and other documents.

Intellectual Property and Copyright Issues

As an educator you will be using information available via various media. It is often confusing to consider the many regulations that apply to others' use of your works and your use of works authored by others. Some of the important concepts about which you should know include copyright, fair use, public domain, plagiarism, and intellectual property rights. In general, it is important to remember that the copyright symbol (©) need not appear for a document or other form of media to be copyrighted. The purpose of copyright law is to protect the ownership of a document, so that the author receives credit for its development and compensation, where applicable.

plagiarism
Representation of the works of another as one's own.

Plagiarism is representing the work of another as your own. This may occur deliberately or because of failure to properly document citations in your work. Not only is this a concern for your work, but you must caution students about plagiarism, as well. Plagiarism has become epidemic in higher education and can be difficult to detect because of the many sources of information available to students. Educational institutions provide definitions of and guidelines for handling plagiarism. Plagiarism is considered to be academic dishonesty and can result in severe disciplinary action, including termination, against students and instructors.

The original copyright law in the United States dates back to 1917 and, as such, does not provide guidance for the use of electronic media. The Digital Millennium Copyright Act of 1998 was enacted to provide regulations for the use of digitally transmitted information. In general, the regulations for the use of copyrighted material are less strict for educational purposes than for personal or proprietary use. This usage is based on the principle of "fair use." However, except for limited circumstances, you must obtain permission, for a fee, to use copyrighted materials from the Copyright Clearance Center. In some cases, educational institutions may have copyright agreements that apply to the use of certain materials. More information on copyright law can be obtained through the Code of Federal Register (CFR) Web site by searching under Title 17, from the Web site of the U.S. Government Printing Office at **www.access.gpo.gov/uscode**, or by going to **www.copyright. gov/title17/**.

There are certain documents, concepts, and phrases that do not require copyright permission. These are considered public domain works. Such works include information that is known to the majority of the public or for whom the original author cannot determined.

The issue of intellectual property rights can become a point of contention between educators and employers. The ownership of documents such as lesson plans and PowerPoint© presentations depends upon the nature of your job and under what circumstances you produced the document. If your job is to provide a professional service, such as teaching, then the documents you create to perform that service can be considered personal work products and most likely belong to you. If you produce a document on your own time, using your own resources, it belongs to you even if you use it in your job. Intellectual property is presently a hot topic in higher education. You can find out more on the Web site of the National Education Association (NEA) at **http://www. nea.org/he/abouthe/intelprop.html**.

Student Conduct and Grievances

It is necessary for program policies to address all information for which you want students to be held responsible. Some of these areas include students' rights and responsibilities, academic integrity, professional conduct, substance use, affirmative-action and equal-opportunity issues, grading policies, penalties for breaches of policy, and grievance procedures.

Academic integrity applies to plagiarism, cheating, falsification of documents, and attempts to reconstruct examination questions for use by that student or by others. Higher-education institutions have policies governing these issues and the steps to be taken regarding them. If you are teaching for a program that is not in an institution of higher education, it will be helpful for you to review the documents used by such institutions as a guide in creating your own policies.

Policies of educational institutions also usually address other issues, such as possession or use of substances and weapons, student rights and responsibilities, and student conduct. Your program policies should refer students to the institutional policies. If your particular program has more stringent requirements than exist at the institutional level, you must specifically address these in the program handbook and/or course policies.

As discussed earlier in the chapter, students may become disgruntled for a number of reasons. Clear policies and documentation of student receipt of policies can go a long way toward heading off student grievances or at least can minimize the chances of the grievance being substantiated. Your program policy must address the student-grievance process. In the event that a student initiates a grievance, you must allow the student to go through the process without fear of retaliation. Thorough documentation of student performance, student-incident reports, and student-counseling sessions will support your actions in the event of a grievance.

Other Areas of Legal Concern to the EMS Educator

Certain other laws regarding pay and workplace issues may pertain to the EMS educator, too. As an employee it is important that you know your rights in the workplace. If you are or will be in a supervisory role, you must be aware of laws pertaining to hiring, firing, work hours, and compensation. You should consult with the human resources staff regarding these issues and follow your employer's published policies. Occupational Safety and Health Administration regulations apply to employee health and safety in educational settings, as they do to other workplaces. In particular, because of the nature of EMS education, you should be aware of guidelines regarding body-substance isolation and the handling of contaminated sharps and other items. You can find additional information on these topics at **www.osha.gov/**. For Internal Revenue Service regulations, search Title 26 of the CFR.

Considerations in Risk Management

Most institutions in which EMS education takes place have a department, or at least an individual, in charge of risk management. Your program should work with this department to minimize the program's

indemnification
A legal exemption from liability for damages.

liability. Risk-management strategies include requirements for student health insurance, safety training, health screening, immunizations, student malpractice insurance, instructor malpractice insurance, instructor health insurance, policies for incidents and exposures, and **indemnification** (compensation for harm or damages) issues between the institution and clinical sites.

Ethics in EMS Education

Ethics are important in both medicine and teaching. In both, we deal with the diversity of people's beliefs, actions, cultures, and behaviors on a daily basis. Professional ethics are a part of the different levels of EMS NSC, meaning there will be a specific lesson on ethics early in your courses. But teaching ethics does not stop there. There will many occasions during case studies and students' discussions of their clinical experiences to provide students with opportunities for ethical problem solving. Your role will be primarily to pose problems and ask questions that facilitate discussion. Your goal is to get students to examine their own beliefs, assumptions, and actions. You must be prepared to handle disagreement among students in a productive manner, because there are many complexities in ethical dilemmas upon which students will not agree, and about which they will feel strongly.

In addition to being prepared to facilitate the development of student ethics, as an educator you will be faced with many situations involving ethics. Fortunately, there are guidelines for the conduct of educators in general, found in the NEA Code of Ethics (Box 3-4), and a specific statement of good practices for EMS educators developed by NAEMSE, found at **http://www.naemse.org/positionpapers/GoodPractices.pdf**.

morals
Principles of right and wrong in human conduct.

values
Things and ideas that people hold as personally important.

ethics
A branch of philosophy that deals with the study of morality; can also be considered to be the specific standards and rules of conduct of a profession.

Ethics, Values, Morality, and Legality

Ethics, morals, values, and laws are all guides for conduct. It can be confusing to distinguish between them; in truth, they are related concepts that overlap to a certain degree in their usage but are distinguished from one another by their definitions. **Morals** are the principles of right and wrong in human conduct. They are largely based in the religious culture of the society and, thus, in Western culture are based on Judeo-Christian values (the common beliefs of Judaism and Christianity). **Values** are the things and ideas that people hold as personally important and are related to morals. In fact, these two concepts are often linked together in the term *moral values*. **Ethics** is a branch of philosophy that deals with the study of morality and can also be considered the specific standards and rules of conduct of a profession. The *laws* of a society are based on

(*continued on page* 39)

Box 3.4

Code of Ethics of the Education Profession

Preamble

The educator, believing in the worth and dignity of each human being, recognizes the supreme importance of the pursuit of truth, devotion to excellence, and the nurture of the democratic principles. Essential to these goals is the protection of freedom to learn and to teach and the guarantee of equal educational opportunity for all. The educator accepts the responsibility to adhere to the highest ethical standards.

The educator recognizes the magnitude of the responsibility inherent in the teaching process. The desire for the respect and confidence of one's colleagues, of students, of parents, and of the members of the community provides the incentive to attain and maintain the highest possible degree of ethical conduct. The Code of Ethics of the Education Profession indicates the aspiration of all educators and provides standards by which to judge conduct.

The remedies specified by the NEA and/or its affiliates for the violation of any provision of this Code shall be exclusive and no such provision shall be enforceable in any form other than the one specifically designated by the NEA or its affiliates.

PRINCIPLE I

Commitment to the Student

The educator strives to help each student realize his or her potential as a worthy and effective member of society. The educator therefore works to stimulate the spirit of inquiry, the acquisition of knowledge and understanding, and the thoughtful formulation of worthy goals.

In fulfillment of the obligation to the student, the educator—

1. Shall not unreasonably restrain the student from independent action in the pursuit of learning.
2. Shall not unreasonably deny the student's access to varying points of view.
3. Shall not deliberately suppress or distort subject matter relevant to the student's progress.
4. Shall make reasonable effort to protect the student from conditions harmful to learning or to health and safety.

5. Shall not intentionally expose the student to embarrassment or disparagement.
6. Shall not on the basis of race, color, creed, sex, national origin, marital status, political or religious beliefs, family, social or cultural background, or sexual orientation, unfairly—

   a. Exclude any student from participation in any program
   b. Deny benefits to any student
   c. Grant any advantage to any student

7. Shall not use professional relationships with students for private advantage.
8. Shall not disclose information about students obtained in the course of professional service unless disclosure serves a compelling professional purpose or is required by law.

PRINCIPLE II

Commitment to the Profession

The education profession is vested by the public with a trust and responsibility requiring the highest ideals of professional service.

In the belief that the quality of the services of the education profession directly influences the nation and its citizens, the educator shall exert every effort to raise professional standards, to promote a climate that encourages the exercise of professional judgment, to achieve conditions that attract persons worthy of the trust to careers in education, and to assist in preventing the practice of the profession by unqualified persons.

In fulfillment of the obligation to the profession, the educator—

1. Shall not in an application for a professional position deliberately make a false statement or fail to disclose a material fact related to competency and qualifications.
2. Shall not misrepresent his/her professional qualifications.
3. Shall not assist any entry into the profession of a person known to be unqualified in respect to character, education, or other relevant attribute.
4. Shall not knowingly make a false statement concerning the qualifications of a candidate for a professional position.
5. Shall not assist a noneducator in the unauthorized practice of teaching.

6. Shall not disclose information about colleagues obtained in the course of professional service unless disclosure serves a compelling professional purpose or is required by law.

7. Shall not knowingly make false or malicious statements about a colleague.

8. Shall not accept any gratuity, gift, or favor that might impair or appear to influence professional decisions or action.

Courtesy NEA. Adopted by the NEA 1975 Representative Assembly.

morals but cannot govern all aspects of human life. Therefore, society relies on morals to guide behaviors that cannot be governed by law. Ethics and morals are obviously closely related. We will discuss both theories of human moral development, which will help you understand students' abilities to solve ethical dilemmas, and the professional ethics guiding education practice.

Moral Development

There are several theories of moral development, which is dependent upon—but not synonymous with—cognitive (intellectual) development. Moral development continues into adulthood and is a contemporary issue in higher education. In fact, the original purpose of higher education was moral development, not intellectual development. Two useful theories of moral development were formulated by Kohlberg (1969) and Rest (1984).

Rest's four-component model of morality (1984) suggests that, rather than just focusing on moral judgment, we must consider moral sensitivity, moral judgment, moral motivation, and moral character. *Moral sensitivity* refers to a person's ability to identify a moral issue in a situation and to consider the effects of various decisions on the well-being of others. This capability depends upon a person's ability to empathize with others. *Moral judgment* is the act of bringing social norms to bear on decisions about possible courses of action that could be taken in a situation. Such norms can include justice, social responsibility, unselfishness, cooperation, keeping promises, and reciprocity of actions. This depends on the person's acquisition of the norms of a particular society. *Moral motivation* refers to a person's ability and willingness to prioritize moral actions over competing values such as avoiding punishment, financial security, career promotion, or disapproval by one's peer group. *Moral character* refers to the psychological strength needed to carry out moral decisions.

ON TARGET According to to Rest (1984) the four components of moral development are moral sensitivity, moral judgment, moral motivation, and moral character.

Kohlberg's (1969) theory of moral judgment consists of three levels of development: preconventional morality, conventional morality, and postconventional morality. In *preconventional morality* a person considers what is "good" or "bad" in terms of his or her individual needs. Good and bad are concrete categories and a thing is either good or bad, in relationship to the needs of the individual. *Conventional morality* is based on beliefs about the importance of maintaining relationships and what it takes to do so. At this level moral behavior is understood as "being nice" to others. Laws are seen as absolutes in terms of regulating "good" and "bad" behaviors in society. *Postconventional morality* is based on conscience or principles. For example, a given law may be recognized as being fair or appropriate in some situations, but not others. The overriding principles include the value of human life, justice, service to others, respect for human differences and dignity, and contribution to the common good.

Many influences affect an individual's moral development. In general, intellectual development is related to moral development such that individuals with the capacity for reflective thinking are much more likely to be able to overcome influences such as parental values, religious teaching, and stereotypes. These individuals can much more easily base decisions on evidence and the situation at hand, rather than on preexisting biases (Guthrie 1996).

Moral Education

The EMS educator can facilitate moral development through role modeling, direct teaching, and experiential techniques. Teachers are role models, whether they intend to be or not. By virtue of their position, students will look to them as models for their own beliefs and behaviors. It is essential that educators keep this in mind in monitoring their own decisions and conduct. In direct teaching, it is important that teachers do not "preach from the pulpit" but instead hold ethical behavior as an ideal to which we all aspire, while recognizing that humans are imperfect beings and will sometimes fall short of ideals. By presenting case studies and discussing students' clinical experiences, the EMS educator can provide questions for reflection on action. Some questions might include, Did you have any emotions or beliefs that were in conflict with respect for human dignity in making the decision to withhold CPR? or Has concern over being confronted by a nurse in the emergency department ever caused you to make a patient uncomfortable with spinal immobilization procedures, even though you knew the mechanism of injury did not call for it? The educator can provide a framework for the interpretation of situations by asking the impact of social norms such as equity and trust in authority on the decision-making process.

Professional Ethics

As discussed previously, the NEA Code of Ethics is given in Box 3-4. The NAEMSE *Statement of Good Practices by EMS Educators in the Discharge of Their Ethical and Professional Responsibilities* is given on the NAEMSE Web site, as mentioned, and is summarized here.

EMS educators are seen as having ethical responsibility to students, colleagues, the profession, and the general public. As educators, we have a powerful influence on students' attitudes about the provider-patient relationship, professional competence, and professional responsibility. We must always keep the intensity of this influence in mind in our teaching. We must strive for excellence in teaching and treat others with civility, respect, and fairness. We must recognize our obligation to evaluate student progress and competence in a valid and impartial manner and must maintain student confidentiality, except where disclosure is required by law.

As professional educators, we have an obligation to communicate information that is valid and unbiased. We have an obligation to construct knowledge of the field through research and publication and to recognize the contributions of others. We are obligated to treat our colleagues with respect; finally, we have a duty to the public to promote excellence in prehospital care through our influence on students and have a responsibility for public education.

Summary

Legal and ethical considerations in EMS and in EMS education often present as complex, ambiguously structured problems. As such, it is imperative that EMS educators have—and impart to their students—an understanding of the principles, guidelines, frameworks, and references available to them in recognizing and solving such problems. There are many sources of information on regulations governing the conduct of EMS education, many of which are provided in this chapter. In guiding ethical conduct in EMS education practice, the NEA Code of Ethics and the NAEMSE statement of good practices serve as guidelines for behavior. In facilitating the moral development of students, the

EMS educator can use role modeling, direct teaching, and experiential activities to raise students' awareness of issues and provide a framework for problem solving.

REVIEW QUESTIONS

1. List three potential areas for EMS educator liability.

2. In your own words, define *educational malpractice*.

3. In what, if any, instance may an educational institution release a student's educational record to a third party?

4. Following ADA, what are the student's obligations in receiving accommodations?

5. In Rest's model of moral development, what does *moral sensitivity* mean?

Institutions, Settings, and Types of Programs

Learning Objectives

Upon completion of this chapter you should be able to

- Compare and contrast the characteristics of the different settings in which the EMS educator may practice.

- Differentiate between primary, refresher, and continuing education.

- Discuss the purposes of traditional classroom, laboratory, clinical, and virtual classroom education.

CASE Study_____

Maria Vasquez has just completed an EMS-Instructor course and is doing an instructor internship with the fire-training academy. She is excited at the prospect of getting a job as an EMS instructor. She is considering applying to a nearby vocational career center that offers EMT-Basic courses, a community college that offers EMT-Basic and paramedic courses as well as a continuing education program, and a trauma center that has paramedic and continuing education programs.

Questions

1. What qualifications is Maria likely to need to work in the trauma center program?

2. What additional credentials might Maria need to work in a community college program?

3. Would working in the vocational school program require any additional credentials?

Introduction

EMS educators function in a variety of institutional and classroom settings and are responsible for different types of programs. Some of the institutional settings include public secondary schools, career centers, hospitals, fire departments, private and municipal ambulance services, government agencies, law-enforcement academies, community colleges, and universities. Within each of these institutions the EMS educator may be involved in **didactic** education, laboratory education, or clinical education. Increasingly, EMS educators are delivering instruction via distance education as well. EMS educators are involved in all levels of EMS education from the pre-EMS level to the paramedic level and may participate in teaching physicians, nurses, physician's assistants, and other types of health-care providers. EMS educators can also play an important role in community health education. As an EMS educator, you may be involved in primary education programs, continuing and refresher education programs, and specialty certification courses, such as Prehospital Trauma Life Support (PHTLS), Advanced Cardiac Life Support (ACLS), Advanced Medical Life Support (AMLS), and Pediatric Advanced Life Support (PALS).

didactic
Instruction or something that is intended to teach. Usually used to refer to classroom, rather than laboratory activities.

KEY TERMS

clinical education, p. 51	distance education, p. 51	secondary education, p. 45
cohort, p. 51	intranet, p. 51	university, p. 46
community college, p. 46	laboratory, p. 50	virtual education, p. 51
continuing education, p. 47	primary education, p. 47	vocational education, p. 44
didactic, p. 44	refresher education, p. 47	

Institutional Settings

vocational education
Education or training specific to one's intended occupation.

Secondary Education and Career Centers

Regulations in some states allow students under the age of 18 to participate in basic life-support-level courses. Therefore, in some states First Responder or EMT courses may be offered through **vocational education** departments in high schools. The requirements for teaching in vocational education programs in the public school system vary from state to state. Area career centers are often operated by the public school system and may include **secondary education** as well as adult education classes for high school completion or vocational training, and career counseling. Even EMS educators who are not involved in secondary and vocational programs are frequently asked to speak to students considering health careers about EMS education and career opportunities. EMS educators are called upon to give talks or presentations to elementary school audiences, too. It is beyond the scope of this chapter to discuss lifespan development, but should you be invited to speak to or teach school-age children or adolescents, it is helpful to review the cognitive and psychosocial developmental characteristics of these age groups in a paramedic text or other relevant source. This can help you anticipate some of the questions you may be asked and formulate age-appropriate answers.

secondary education
Education in middle and high schools.

PEARLS *Some states require a secondary school teaching license or vocational teaching license or certificate to teach in high schools or vocational schools.*

Hospitals

Many hospitals have roles for EMS educators. Some hospitals offer a full range of primary and continuing education courses in EMS and have an EMS education department. These departments may operate as part of a hospital-based ambulance service, the emergency department or trauma center, or as a part of the education or human resources development department of the hospital. Some hospital-based programs are affiliated with institutions of higher education that provide college credit or advanced standing in college programs to the students of the hospital-based program. An additional benefit of such an arrangement is the availability of academic resources, and sometimes student services, through the college or university. These resources, whether provided by the hospital or affiliated institution, are critical components of a quality educational program. The availability of these resources is examined closely as part of accreditation processes.

The Fire Service, EMS, Public Safety, and Government Agencies

The EMS educator can fit into these settings in a variety ways. In such settings EMS education may operate through a training academy or training department. The EMS educator may be part of the "career" side of such agencies, or can be a civilian employee. Many such agencies outsource their EMS education functions to hospitals, colleges, or universities. Thus, the EMS educator in these institutions may teach in the public safety and governmental sector as well.

The Community College

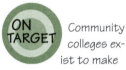

The EMS Agenda for the Future (NHTSA 1996) calls for EMS education to be regarded as an endeavor worthy of academic credit. The 1998 Paramedic NSC (NHTSA 1998) calls for competency in writing, math, and anatomy and physiology at a postsecondary level as prerequisites to paramedic programs. Although there is no mandate for EMS programs to be offered through postsecondary institutions, doing so makes sense. In fact, there are many EMS programs operating through **community colleges** throughout the nation. EMS courses may be offered as electives or as part of certificate or associate degree programs. EMS programs in community colleges may be part of an academic school or department, such as nursing or health sciences, or may be offered through a continuing-education division of the college. The credentials for teaching at the community college level vary and may be different according to whether you are classified as adjunct faculty or staff or regular faculty or staff. These credentials may be required by the state's board of higher education or may be requirements of the employer.

The University

The **university** differs from the community college in its mission and the levels of education offered. Community colleges exist to make higher education widely available, and offer certificates and associate degrees. Colleges generally offer bachelor's degrees but may also offer associate degrees. Universities have active research programs and offer both undergraduate (bachelor's) degree programs and graduate (master's and doctoral) degree programs. There are currently 13 EMS programs in the United States offering bachelor's degrees (Lindstrom and Losavio 2004).

Universities have high standards for the credentials of regular faculty and usually require a minimum of a master's degree. EMS is fairly unique in this requirement, because faculty appointments generally are made only to individuals with doctoral degrees. There is an informal rule in academia that an instructor must hold a degree at least one level higher than the degree program in which he or she is teaching. Master's level instructors are frequently doctoral students working as teaching or graduate assistants. EMS programs at the university level are a fairly new phenomenon, which means that the "terminal degree" in EMS at the present time is the bachelor's degree. Although many individuals in EMS hold master's degrees and even doctoral degrees, these degrees, with very few exceptions, are not in EMS.

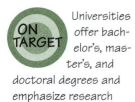

Universities offer bachelor's, master's, and doctoral degrees and emphasize research activities.

Universities, particularly those with a medical school and affiliated teaching hospital, offer tremendous resources to EMS students. Whereas many institutions without medical schools or large nursing or health sciences programs have a medical or health sciences collection in the main library, medical schools have separate medical libraries. Other benefits can include involvement of physician faculty and gross anatomy and cadaver labs.

Types of Courses and Programs

Primary Education Programs

primary education
In EMS, preservice education.

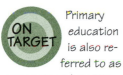

Primary education is also referred to as preservice education.

In EMS, when we refer to **primary education**, we mean the courses that lead to certification at one of the levels recognized by NHTSA or state regulatory agencies, such as First Responder, EMT-Basic, etc. These are sometimes called *preservice education courses*. These programs require approval of the state regulatory agency and must comply with specified curricular guidelines, instructor qualifications, equipment requirements, class-size limitations, and student-entry requirements.

All levels of national standard EMS curricula can be found at **www.nhtsa.dot.gov/people/injury/ems**. It is important to remember that your state EMS regulatory agency may require additional educational modules or restrict the content of the NSC. You must be certain to use the curriculum required by your state.

continuing education
Professional educational courses offered for the purpose of acquiring new knowledge and skills.

refresher education
Educational offerings designed to cover specific content areas included in primary education.

Continuing Education

There are state and NREMT educational requirements for continued certification and reregistration. These requirements may refer to either refresher education or **continuing education**. Although people tend to use the term continuing education as if it is synonymous with refresher education, the terms refer to different educational concepts. **Refresher education** refers to the process of reexposure to primary education content to either reestablish or maintain minimum competency. Continuing education, which has a number of variations on its name (see Box 4-1), refers to the process of learning additional knowledge or skills to enhance practice beyond minimum competency as well as remaining up to date on changes in knowledge and practice.

Box 4-1

Continuing-Education Abbreviations

Continuing Education	CE
Continuing Professional Education	CPE
Continuing Medical Education	CME
Continuing Education Unit	CEU
Continuing Education Credit	CEC

Although the concept of lifelong learning is certainly not limited to an individual's career needs, continuing education is related to lifelong learning.

Although it is called continuing education, what many states require is refresher education. The requirements for reregistration with the NREMT can be found on its Web site at **www.nremt.org**. Many state EMS agencies list their recertification requirements on their Web sites, too. The practice of continuing education (and refresher education) comes with many challenges. The difficulty for the EMS educator is in presenting material that many of the attendees have heard over and over again. Attendees are understandably bored and, in some cases, hostile about being mandated to attend a course that does not make good use of their time. It is not uncommon for the educator to be the recipient of the attendees' frustrated complaints and, at times, disruptive behavior. True continuing education, even when expertly presented, may not be relevant to the needs of the audience. Needs analysis is an essential, but often overlooked, part of continuing education. If you find yourself offering the same continuing-education class on multiple occasions, it may also become a challenge to remain fresh and enthusiastic in the classroom.

Specialty Certification Courses

Currently the specialty certification courses relevant to EMS require an instructor course specific to that particular program. Although these instructor courses are not comprehensive, they do provide specific information on the administrative requirements for conducting the course. Many employers require EMS educators to maintain instructor status in CPR, ACLS, a trauma certification course such as Prehospital Trauma Life Support (PHTLS) or Basic Trauma Life Support (BTLS), and sometimes Pediatric Advanced Life Support (PALS). Box 4-2 lists some of the certificate courses for which EMS educators may wish to attain instructor status.

Box4-2

Specialty Certification Courses

AMERICAN HEART ASSOCIATION

www.americanheart.org   ACLS   Advanced Cardiac Life Support

CPR   Cardiopulmonary Resuscitation

PALS   Pediatric Advanced Life Support

AMERICAN ACADEMY OF PEDIATRICS

www.aap.org/

www.aap.org/nrp/nrpmain.html   NRP   Neonatal Resuscitation Program

http://www.peppsite.com/   PEPP   Pediatric Emergencies for Prehospital Providers

http://www.aap.org/apls/aplsmain.htm   APLS   Advanced Pediatric Life Support

NATIONAL ASSOCIATION OF EMTS

www.naemt.org

http://phtls.org/   PHTLS   Prehospital Trauma Life Support

AMLS   Advanced Medical Life Support

PPC   Pediatric Prehospital Care

BASIC TRAUMA LIFE SUPPORT INTERNATIONAL

http://www.btls.org/   BTLS   Basic Trauma Life Support

AMERICAN RED CROSS

http://www.redcross.org/services/hss/courses/   First Aid, CPR, and AED training

NATIONAL SAFETY COUNCIL

http://www.nsc.org/train/ec/   First Aid, CPR, AED, and Blood-borne Pathogens training

Teaching-Learning Settings

EMS educators may teach in a variety of teaching-learning settings, including classroom, laboratory, clinical, and, increasingly, virtual settings. Each of these settings has specific considerations. Content expertise and speaking ability do not necessarily translate into effective classroom teaching. Teaching in the laboratory requires special knowledge related to psychomotor skills and integration of knowledge. Clinical teaching, too, has its special considerations. Providing courses via various media methods involves many skills beyond the technical expertise needed to put the course together. Methods for teaching in each of these areas are covered in detail in later chapters. The purpose here is to provide an overview of teaching-learning settings.

The Traditional Classroom

The term traditional classroom is used here to mean the customary face-to-face interaction in courses where we expect lecture and discussion. The primary purpose of the instructor-student interaction in this setting is to deliver information and teach cognitive skills. Although we most often think of lecture as the primary means of content delivery in this setting, we can use a variety of teaching-learning methods in the traditional classroom setting, such as lecture-discussion, case studies, and small group activities. A certain amount of affective learning can take place in the classroom, too, through case studies, discussions, and role-play. Both the instructor and students have roles and responsibilities in the traditional classroom setting, and both must come prepared to result in an effective teaching-learning transaction. Students must do their readings and other assignments prior to class and come prepared to both ask and answer questions and contribute to discussion and in-class activities. As an instructor, you will need to come armed with educational process knowledge and content expertise.

The Laboratory

laboratory
A place for practice, observation, or testing.

The **laboratory,** or lab as most students and instructors call it, is the setting in which instructors assist students in learning the steps of psychomotor skills and under what circumstances their use is indicated. This process requires the integration of cognitive, psychomotor, and affective learning. Once the steps of a skill have been learned, the laboratory is a place for integrated scenario-based practice. The circumstances for teaching in the laboratory require a lower instructor-to-student ratio than in the classroom and active participation on the part of the students. In many cases there are individuals who work primarily as lab instructors, usually on a part-time or volunteer basis. Laboratory education is as critical as classroom education, but it is sometimes assumed that any good practitioner can teach skills. In addition to being able to expertly perform skills, lab instructors must understand the educational processes important to teaching psychomotor skills in order to be effective lab instructors.

The Clinical Setting

clinical education
The portion of a health sciences student's education that takes place in the service setting and involves supervised performance of job tasks.

Clinical education takes place in the service setting and is where students continue to learn through supervised performance of duties in a real-world setting. It requires the application of didactic, psychomotor, and affective learning and reflection on experiences. Clinical education includes both in-hospital and out-of-hospital experiences. Effective clinical education requires preceptors who are knowledgeable about learning and who are willing to work through clinical problem solving with students rather than taking over a situation as soon as a student shows hesitation. Clinical educators must direct students toward appropriate experiences and ask questions to promote critical thinking and reflection on experience. Although instructor certification is not required of clinical preceptors, clinical preceptors must be educated about their roles and responsibilities as preceptors. Too often, this part of EMS education is neglected.

intranet
A computer communication system linking computers on the same network.

The Virtual Classroom

distance education
An educational program offered through a medium other than face-to-face contact between students and instructor. Includes Internet-based education as well as televised broadcasts, CD-ROMs, and self-study modules.

Both primary and continuing education may take place via Internet-based programs, CD-ROMs, and televised broadcasts. Many colleges and universities have Web-based courseware licenses for platforms (such as Blackboard™) that are available to faculty and staff to construct distance courses or to supplement traditional classroom learning. Other large organizations may have an **intranet** that can be used for education. Although **distance education** is limited to cognitive domain teaching and learning, it offers students the flexibility to work around their schedules and other obligations. Many students in rural areas would otherwise have very restricted access to education. There are educational principles that must be applied to construct such courses well, but it is, unfortunately, not uncommon for poorly constructed programs to be marketed. Many students in distance education feel isolated and miss the **cohort** feeling that occurs when people meet face to face over several weeks, months, or semesters. Well-constructed distance education, or **virtual education**, programs incorporate measures that help minimize these feelings.

cohort
A group with chronological commonality, such as a group of individuals who move through a program of studies together.

virtual education
Distance education, especially by Internet.

Summary

Whether full-time or part-time, there is a variety of opportunities for EMS educators. As an EMS educator you can be involved in teaching primary education, continuing-education, and specialty certification courses. There may be additional credentials necessary for teaching specialty courses. Options for employment include public safety agencies, hospitals, secondary and vocational schools, community colleges, and universities. In some settings, college credits or a degree may be required, as may a criminal background investigation, in addition to state EMS educator certification. Teaching in the classroom, lab, clinical setting, and virtually all require particular knowledge.

REVIEW QUESTIONS

1. List at least four settings in which an EMS educator may find work.

2. Explain the difference between continuing education and refresher education.

3. How do community colleges, colleges, and universities differ from each other?

4. In addition to EMS instructor certification or recognition, what other types of credentials may be required by employers?

5. Differentiate the purposes and activities of didactic, laboratory, and clinical education.

Qualities, Competencies, Roles, and Responsibilities of EMS Educators

Learning Objectives

Upon completion of this chapter you should be able to

- Communicate the affective traits and professional competencies required of an EMS educator.

- Detail the roles and responsibilities of EMS educators.

- Differentiate between the roles and responsibilities of primary and secondary EMS instructors.

- Explain the importance of continuing professional development in EMS education.

- Identify mechanisms through which continuing professional development may be undertaken.

- Describe an EMS educator's relationship with students, assistant instructors, peers, the program director, and the medical director.

- Access educational resources and research.

- Define the terminology of educational practice introduced in this chapter.

Todd LeBeau has been a paramedic for 7 years and has been a part-time secondary instructor for the EMT-Basic program at the area community college for the past 2 years. He is respected as an instructor and his instructor peers consider him to be a role model. Yesterday Pam Mikels, the program director, asked Todd if he would be interested in being a full-time primary instructor for the program. Todd knows that his responsibilities in the program will be different, but he doesn't know exactly what will be expected of him. Todd makes an appointment to meet with Pam to discuss the position.

Questions

1. In what ways could Todd's role as a primary instructor differ from his role as a secondary instructor?
2. What questions should Todd ask Pam about the position?
3. What qualities make an instructor a good role model for other instructors as well as for students?

Introduction

Arranging conditions conducive to learning involves artistry, a specific body of knowledge, and a distinct set of abilities. Although some individuals seem to be "born teachers" because of their intuitive or artful approach, there is a specific body of knowledge in education, for which research evidence is abundant, that is required for effective teaching. The art of teaching can be developed, and the expertise and abilities can be learned. The practice of EMS education requires particular affective qualities and professional proficiencies as the basis for effectively assuming the roles played by educators and fulfilling the responsibilities associated with those roles. As you begin practice you will need to understand the common terminology of educational practice in order to communicate with your peers and continue learning about education. This chapter introduces some of the terms used in the professional practice of education. The purpose of this chapter is to discuss the traits and abilities needed by EMS educators and to define their roles and responsibilities.

Terminology

Before proceeding with the information in this and later chapters, it is necessary to establish a common understanding of the terminology that is used. Some of the terms are specific to EMS education, and others are used more generally in education and other fields in the social sciences. Understanding the specialized terminology of a field of practice is essential to communicating with colleagues and taking advantage of opportunities for further professional development.

primary instructor
The instructor with ultimate responsibility for a course and who generally does most of the teaching of that course.

secondary instructor
A less-experienced instructor with less responsibility for course coordination.

Primary and Secondary Instructors

The NHTSA guidelines for EMS instructors (2002) differentiate between **primary instructors** and **secondary instructors**. According to these guidelines, a primary instructor possesses appropriate academic and/or allied health credentials, has an understanding of principles and theories of education, and has an adequate amount of teaching experience to provide quality instruction. A secondary instructor differs in that he or she has limited teaching experience. The secondary instructor assists in instruction but is not ultimately responsible for the overall administration of the course.

ON TARGET Secondary instructors have not yet accumulated the degree of teaching experiences expected of primary instructors.

Cohort

The term **cohort** is not unique to education and is used in other fields to describe a collection of people who have some chronological commonality as a group. The term is often used in research to describe a group being studied—for example, a group of individuals who were all born in the same year. In education we refer to a cohort as a group of students who are attending a class or classes together and move through their program of studies in the same time frame.

Class

The meaning of the term class varies slightly, depending upon the context in which it is used. A **class** may be a block of instruction delivered on a single occasion. For example, a lecture on the medical-legal aspects of EMS from 7:00 P.M. to 9:00 P.M. on Tuesday is a class. The term session can also be used for this purpose. For example, a semester-long course may consist of 15 classes, or sessions. The second way class is used in the educational setting is to refer to the group of students attending a class session.

Program

The term *program* also has two different meanings, depending on context. A **program** can refer to the organized structure of an educational offering that has multiple units, blocks, or modules of instruction, such as a paramedic program, EMT-Basic program, and so forth. Program is also used to mean the organized entity that designs, develops, and delivers education. For example, there may be an EMS program in a university that consists of the personnel and resources needed to conduct educational offerings.

Event

An **event** is an educational session that occurs on one occasion, such as a presentation on detecting academic dishonesty offered to the faculty and staff by the director of the academic integrity office at a college or university.

Professional Qualities of the Adult Educator

The desirable general characteristics of EMS educators are those that apply to all adult educators. These characteristics are quite similar to the professional behaviors expected of paramedics. The EMS educator possesses integrity and honesty, values lifelong learning, and is empathetic and compassionate, self-motivated, professional in appearance, self-confident, able to communicate clearly, effective in time management, an advocate of teamwork, diplomatic, respectful, knowledgeable about the subject matter being taught, and an advocate for the student. Beyond being able to list these qualities, it is important to be able to carry them out in practice.

Honesty and Integrity

honesty
Truthful, fair, sincere, of good reputation.

integrity
Adherence to a standard of values.

Honesty and integrity relate to ethics and moral development, as discussed in Chapter 3. **Honesty** can be considered in many forms. Being honest means to act truthfully and without deceit. It also refers to sincerity, lack of pretension, and respectability. **Integrity** in this context refers to the quality of adhering to morals, values, and ethics. So as such, integrity is related to, but is much broader than, honesty. Empathy and compassion are also moral concepts based on the ability to see and understand situations from the perspectives of others and to treat others in a humane manner.

Self-Motivation

intrinsic
Something that is inherent or situated within a person or thing.

self-motivation
Having the incentive to take action.

Being self-motivated is a redundancy, because all motivation is **intrinsic** to the individual; all motivation is **self-motivation.** Motivation is a desire to act in order to meet some unmet need, whether it is physical, social, emotional, or intellectual. Teaching is a rewarding experience that fulfills some of the needs of the educator. This is the impetus behind the actions of the educator. Often people disagree about the intrinsic nature of motivation. By way of illustration, consider that in most circumstances adults enter educational programs because they see the program as a way of meeting one or more needs. Try to imagine yourself being sent for mandatory training in something you have no interest in, are afraid of, or find distasteful. You may take action to get through or get out of the situation, but the need to get out of an unpleasant experience is your motivation, rather than the motivation to learn. This is an important concept in dealing with students, too. In some instances the educator can help students see avenues of action to meet their needs, can demonstrate how needs can be met through becoming an EMS provider, or can assist in removing barriers to realizing motivation. In other cases, when students are mandated to enroll in an educational program in which they are not interested, it creates a difficult situation. As much as you probably think EMS is a great field of practice, others may not see it that way. This is an instance in which empathy should come into play—again, imagine yourself being mandated to do something which has no appeal to you.

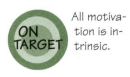
All motivation is intrinsic.

Professional Appearance

Regardless of your expertise as an educator, your credibility will suffer if your appearance does not convey professionalism. There is some variability in what is considered appropriate dress in an educational setting. It is important to consider the body of students and their expectations, the culture of the organization for which you work, and what kind of teaching you will be involved in. At times it is appropriate to wear a uniform, whereas in other circumstances a suit may be correct for the situation. In some situations "dress casual" such as khaki slacks and a polo shirt is the best choice. You need to exercise judgment in selecting appropriate attire. Consider whether you are speaking to a community group, lecturing to a class you have been working with for several weeks, teaching lab skills, or providing clinical supervision. In all circumstances, good hygiene and grooming are expected.

Self-Confidence

self-confidence
A person's belief in his or her competence.

Self-confidence, the belief that you are competent to carry out the duties of your role, is important. The message of even the most knowledgeable individual may be lost if students perceive doubt or nervousness in the speaker's verbal or nonverbal communications. Self-confidence is warranted when you are prepared for your task. Avoid being overly confident or smug; it will negatively impact your relationship with students and colleagues.

Effective Communication

Written and verbal communication skills are vital to the educational process. A good portion of what we do is conveying and receiving information. Students expect that their instructors will have good writing and speaking skills—that the instructor can write clear directions for homework, exams, and projects and present lecture material in a clear, logical manner. Factors such as poor grammar, misspellings, and mispronunciations detract from the credibility of the instructor.

Time Management

There are many facets of time management for the EMS educator. You will need to get an idea of how long it takes to prepare for a class, to write lesson plans, and other preparatory activities. These activities will be quite time consuming at first, but you will become more proficient with experience. It will also take a measure of experience before you get an idea of how much material or how much lab activity fits into a given time period. Instructors must pay attention to the need for breaks during instructional activities as well. All this must be done in addition to managing the other activities of your career and life!

Teamwork Orientation

A collaborative or teamwork approach to teaching enriches the educational experience of students by bringing in the perspectives and strengths of colleagues. Ideally, this collaborative approach brings together the didactic, laboratory, and clinical components of the educational program to offer an integrated program of studies. Teamwork is important in student interactions as well, and the adult educator must create an atmosphere of collaboration and teamwork among students, rather than promoting competition between them.

Diplomacy and Respect

diplomacy
Tact in dealing with people.

respect
To show regard or consideration for someone or something.

It is not unusual for students to challenge their instructors regarding class policies, grading issues, or accuracy of content. In addition, there will occasionally be students whose classroom behavior detracts from the quality of the educational environment. These situations, and others, require the use of diplomacy and respect. **Diplomacy** is the ability to use tact in dealing with others, whereas **respect** conveys the willingness to show consideration for others. Respect is a bit broader than diplomacy and includes not just what is said and how, but also such things as counseling students in private and having regard for their dignity and self-esteem. Diplomacy and respect extend not only to interactions with students, but also to what is conveyed to students about, for example, actions of preceptors, institutional authorities, competing programs, and so forth.

Lifelong Learning

lifelong learning
A process of continuing growth and development in knowledge, skills, and character.

Although it seems commonsense, it bears mentioning that educators should value **lifelong learning** for themselves and others. After all, education is our business. Even so, we often put our own personal growth on hold to deal with other priorities. Continued personal growth allows individuals to express their potential and attain achievements in a variety of areas. Continuing professional development, both in content areas and educational process expertise, increases feelings of competence and is an investment in your career. Box 5-1 lists journals useful in professional development of the adult educator. Box 5-2 lists professional organizations that provide resources for continuing professional development in education.

 PEARLS You should read at least one professional journal in adult education or human resources development on a regular basis in order to keep abreast of the latest research and theoretical developments in adult learning.

Box 5-1

Selected Journals for Professional Development

Adult Learning

Adults Learning

Chronicle of Higher Education

Community College Review

International Journal of Lifelong Learning

Journal of Continuing Education in the Health Professions

Journal of Educational Psychology

Journal of Moral Education

New Directions for Adult & Continuing Education

Nursing Education Perspectives

Studies in the Education of Adults

Quarterly Review of Distance Education

Box 5-2

Resource Organizations for Professional Development

American Association for Adult and Continuing Education	www.AAACE.org
American Council on Education	www.acenet.edu
American Society for Training and Development	ww.astd.org
Educational Information Resources Center (ERIC) Clearinghouse on Adult, Career, and Vocational Education	http://ericacve.org
National Association of EMS Educators	www.naemse.org
National Education Association	www.nea.org
United States Department of Education	www.ed.gov/

Content Knowledge

As educators we have an obligation to be knowledgeable about the subject matter that we teach. This does not mean that paramedics should approach topics in the same depth required for physicians, but they must have the knowledge of a highly competent paramedic. Part of an instructor's authority comes from his or her *greater* knowledge and experience in the subject, not from knowing everything there is to know about a topic. Once you have conveyed the subject matter in the depth and breadth appropriate to the curriculum and goals of the program, your obligation to the student who wants to know more is to be able to suggest resources from which the student can gain additional knowledge about the topic. It is somewhat disconcerting when it turns out that one of your students has a degree in neurobiology, physics, law, or some other area that bears on parts of the curriculum. In adult education this is not only to be expected, but also respected. The student should be encouraged to contribute his expertise to the learning of his classmates.

Student Advocacy

advocate
To speak in favor of or support.

Finally, student advocacy is expected of the EMS educator. An **advocate** is a person who supports the causes of another. One clear example of this is negotiating with clinical sites to allow students to perform skills rather than only observing skills. Other examples are inviting employers to discuss career opportunities with students, and writing recommendations for students.

Roles and Responsibilities of Primary and Secondary Instructors

Primary and Secondary Instructors

The term *primary instructor* is used to differentiate the greater roles and responsibilities of the instructor who has the most accountability for a program or course from those of instructors who assist in the classroom. In some areas the primary instructor is referred to as a lead instructor, or instructor of record. Secondary instructors are sometimes called support, or adjunct, instructors. An instructor with minimal teaching experience will serve as a secondary instructor before acting as a primary instructor. Instructors who are primary instructors in other situations may take on the role of secondary instructor in a particular course. The distinction between the two has more to do with roles and responsibilities than it does with seniority, rank, or other credentials.

Roles and Responsibilities

role
A function or position.

responsibility
Accountability or reliability.

The terms roles and responsibilities are often used interchangeably, but they are distinct. A **role** is a function or position. The function or position may be reflected by a job title, such as Adjunct Instructor, or may be a function within a job. For example, a person whose job title is EMS Instructor may take on the role of clinical coordinator. **Responsibilities** are the duties performed within a given role. The clinical coordinator may have responsibilities such as tracking clinical affiliation agreements and sending student schedules to clinical sites.

Roles and Responsibilities of the Primary Instructor

The primary instructor may play roles at both program and course levels. At the program level the primary instructor may have administrative responsibilities, such as publishing or distributing a schedule of courses and ordering supplies. The exact responsibilities differ from institution to institution. Roles of the primary instructor include course administrator, course coordinator, liaison with the medical director and stakeholders, counselor, instructor, mentor, and evaluator.

Responsibilities of the Course Administrator
Administrative duties include completing course paperwork, such as applications for approval by the appropriate regulatory body, end-of-course reports, and submitting grades. The course administrator may also be responsible for maintaining appropriate student documentation, such as copies of CPR cards, certification cards, proof of high school graduation, and criminal background checks. Administrators should develop a mechanism by which they can avoid directly handling or keeping copies of student health documentation. The administrator may also be responsible for maintaining other course and student documents.

Responsibilities of the Course Coordinator
As the course coordinator, the EMS educator performs such tasks as preparing the course syllabus, scheduling classrooms, scheduling guest instructors, ensuring equipment and supplies are available, and scheduling

special events, such as off-site classes in rope rescue or extrication. In this capacity the primary instructor may be involved in developing course policies and evaluating the course. The course coordinator is generally the first point of contact for student grievances and disciplinary issues.

Course Liaison

The primary instructor is likely to be the point of contact for questions about the course, such as inquiries from clinical sites (unless there is a separate clinical coordinator). He or she will also communicate with the medical director for the purposes of keeping the medical director advised of student progress, reporting clinical issues, and requesting his or her participation in teaching and student evaluation.

Responsibilities as Counselor and Mentor

In this role the EMS educator will provide educational and career guidance to students. Students often wish to speak to the instructor about academic issues, schedule issues, job seeking, and other issues. The instructor must also take initiative to counsel students on cognitive and affective development. It is not unusual for students to present personal problems to the instructor, such as relationship difficulties and mental and physical health issues. As an instructor, it is essential that you know your limitations in dealing with such issues. In general it is best to ask the student if he or she is sure he or she wants to speak with you about a personal situation, listen empathetically and nonjudgmentally to the student's concerns, and limit your advice to a recommendation to seek the assistance of someone qualified to help with the problem. Under no circumstances should you become personally involved with the student's situation. Of course, what the student shares with you is confidential.

You may also be either formally or informally involved with mentoring newer instructors as they develop and gain experience. This can include answering questions, asking how things are going, and performing peer evaluations of teaching and instructional activities.

Responsibilities in Evaluation

Evaluation is an ongoing process that begins in the program- or course-planning stage. As a primary instructor you may be responsible for both student and program evaluation. In both instances it is necessary to solicit data both formally and informally in a time frame that allows for modification if necessary. Tasks may include writing or compiling test items, constructing homework assignments, and designing evaluation forms to obtain student feedback. The primary instructor is normally responsible for grading and maintaining records of academic performance. Evaluation may reveal the need for student remediation. In such cases, it is necessary to collect more data from the student to find out his or her study habits and what he or she feels is the difficulty. From this point, the instructor and student will develop a plan of remediation and continued assessment.

Responsibilities Common to Primary and Secondary Instructors

Some responsibilities are common to both primary and secondary EMS instructors. These responsibilities tend to involve the management of specific sections of a course rather than the overall direction of the course. An overview of these responsibilities is provided here to present the big picture of instructor responsibilities, but each is covered in more detail in other chapters.

Classroom Management

Classroom-management tasks include keeping the class on schedule, managing the classroom environment, monitoring the effectiveness of instruction, and managing student attendance. It is important to keep the class on schedule by starting on time, managing breaks, and ending on time, as well as by managing student discussion and delivering instruction in the time allotted. However, if in a given class session you feel that the information was not properly covered or that students did not understand the material, as a secondary instructor you should consult with the primary instructor about the possibility of altering the course schedule in the interest of the students. It is important that the EMS instructor manage the physical classroom environment as well as the learning environment. This includes taking steps to assure adequate lighting, temperature control, seating, and writing surfaces. The learning environment is managed by setting the tone of the teaching-learning exchange. Students should feel safe in asking questions and offering comments, and disruptive situations must be addressed.

Monitoring the effectiveness of instruction is related to keeping the class on schedule and to the need for instructors to be flexible in their approach to subjects. You will need to observe the facial expressions of the students and solicit feedback on their understanding. This should be done frequently so that time is not wasted presenting material that cannot be understood because an essential concept was missed early on. Daily classroom management also includes taking and recording student attendance, including tardiness, failure to return from breaks, and leaving early. In most cases there are requirements that students spend a minimum number of hours in the classroom, making documentation of attendance an important part of compliance with institutional, program, and/or regulatory requirements.

Evaluation and Feedback

Evaluation and feedback are important parts of effective instruction and continuous quality improvement of the educational program. Informal student evaluation takes place through continuous observations of student understanding and performance. This can include looking for puzzled expressions on students' faces and asking questions about course content throughout instruction. Formal student evaluation is planned and uses well-constructed quizzes, exams, and assignments to obtain information about student performance and effectiveness of instruction. Program evaluation can also be formal or informal. It can consist of open discussion with students about whether or not the program is meeting their needs as well as it can or can be formal data collection from students and employers on various aspects of the program. When evaluating students it is important to provide feedback as quickly as possible, usually by the next class session.

Managing Grievances and Discipline

Managing discipline problems and responding to student grievances is an unpleasant task and often makes instructors uncomfortable. Unacceptable behaviors by one or more students must be addressed in fairness to the other students. Failing to address unacceptable behaviors leads to a decrease in respect for the instructor and an overall deterioration of the learning environment. Most disciplinary issues can wait until a break when you can talk to a student in private. In some cases, the behavior must be addressed on the spot. Most times students realize their behavior was not appropriate and are apologetic for the disruption. Occasionally students become defensive and argumentative when confronted with the situation. You must know the program policies related to disciplinary issues, including whom to involve and what action to take. Student grievances can occur for many reasons and in most cases should be referred to the instructor closest to the issue. For example, if a student complains to you about a cardiology quiz given by another instructor, the student should be directed to that instructor. If, however, the complaint involves issues such as sexual harassment, program policies should dictate to whom the complaint should be referred.

Course Documentation and Records

There are a variety of sources of regulations regarding record keeping and documentation. Regulations can be from state EMS agencies, the educational institution, and accreditation agencies. Some of the types of documents that must be generated and maintained include attendance rosters, grade reports, clinical competency reports, disciplinary action reports, student conference and counseling reports, and course correspondence.

Regulations vary as to the format in which the records must be maintained and how the security of the records must be ensured. Recall that FERPA guidelines apply to who may access student records and under what conditions. Guidelines also apply to the length of time records must be maintained.

Planning and Delivering Instruction

As a classroom instructor you are responsible for preparing lesson plans and instructional materials and delivering instruction suited to the material being covered. This requires planning, time management, good communication skills, content knowledge, and skill in using the appropriate audio-visual equipment. You also take attendance, assign and collect homework, and administer quizzes and exams. Preparing lesson plans and delivering instruction are core responsibilities of the EMS instructor. Regardless of how other roles and responsibilities are distributed, all instructors are involved in teaching in the classroom, lab, and/or clinical setting. There are numerous considerations in both preparing lesson plans and instruction. These are addressed in later chapters.

Professional Attributes and Skill Sets

The NHTSA guidelines for EMS instructors specify 10 professional attributes and skill sets for EMS instructors. These qualities and abilities are expressed as criteria, for which there are cognitive and affective developmental targets, referred to in the guidelines as goals, and specific performance outcomes, or terminal performance objectives.

Criterion One

EMS educators must understand the essential concepts and tools of inquiry of the EMS levels and content areas they teach. This understanding is necessary to the educator's purpose of creating meaningful learning experiences. In order to create such experiences the EMS educator must strive toward the following goals.

Cognitive Development

- Understand the major concepts, assumptions, debates, processes of inquiry, and body of knowledge central to the disciplines he or she teaches.
- Understand how the adult learner's conceptual frameworks, or schemata, can positively and negatively impact learning.
- Relate the knowledge of the discipline to related subject areas and clinical practice.

Affective Development

- Recognize that EMS subject matter is not a static body of facts but is complex and changing in nature.
- Seek to maintain a current base of knowledge.
- Appreciate multiple perspectives and help the adult learner understand the learning process.
- Convey enthusiasm for the subject matter.
- Be committed to life-long learning.

Performance Outcomes

- Use multiple representations and explanations of concepts to link new material to the learner's previous experience and existing cognitive framework.
- Present differing theories, methods of inquiry, and ways of deriving knowledge.
- Evaluate teaching resources and curriculum materials for their usefulness in a given teaching-learning situation.
- Develop and use curricula that encourage the learner to critically examine subject matter and to view subject matter from different perspectives.

interdisciplinary
A mutual or reciprocal relationship between areas of study.

- Create **interdisciplinary** learning experiences that allow the learner to integrate knowledge and skills from a variety of subject areas.

Criterion Two

The EMS educator understands the processes and conditions of adult learning and uses this knowledge to support the intellectual, professional, and personal development of the learner. The following goals and outcomes are related to this endeavor.

Cognitive Development

- Understand the learning process as construction of knowledge, acquisition of skills, and development of values.
- Select the instructional strategies that draw on the principles of adult learning.
- Respond to the influence of the learner's physical, social, emotional, moral, and cognitive development on the learning process.
- Understand the relationship between the cognitive, affective, and psychomotor domains of learning.

Affective Development
- Appreciate individual variations in learning and development.
- Respect the diversity of talents and experiences of adult learners.
- Facilitate growth of the learner based on assessment of strengths and weaknesses.

Performance Outcomes
- Consider individual and group performance in the delivery of instruction to meet cognitive, affective, and psychomotor learning needs.
- Assist the learner in reflection on experiences and facilitate linkage of new concepts to existing knowledge.
- Provide opportunities for active engagement of the learner in the learning process.
- Encourage the adult learner to assume responsibility for learning and performance.

Criterion Three

The EMS educator understands differences in learning styles and creates learning experiences that appeal to different styles of learning. Working toward the following goals will assist in the development of this competency.

Cognitive Development
- Match instructional approaches to learning styles.
- Understand physical and psychological sources of interference with learning, including sensory impairments, learning disabilities, and physical and mental challenges.
- Understand issues related to cultural diversity in education.

Affective Development
- Persist in helping all students achieve success.
- Encourage learners to pursue excellence in individual development.
- Respect the uniqueness of each student and his or psychosocial background.
- Strive to make the learner feel valued.

Performance Outcomes
- Select instructional methods appropriate to the learners' learning styles, strengths, and needs.

- Seek assistance in providing accommodations to learners with special needs.
- Facilitate the formation of a learning community in the classroom.

Criterion Four

The EMS educator understands and uses instructional strategies that promote learners' development of higher-order thinking, problem-solving ability, and affective and psychomotor development. To do this, the following enabling goals are necessary.

Cognitive Development
- Use an understanding of the different levels of learning within each domain of learning to select strategies appropriate to the level of learning required.
- Understand the appropriate uses, advantages, and disadvantages of various instructional strategies.
- Use educational, human, and technological resources to enhance the learning process.

Affective Development
- Value the development of adult learners' critical thinking, problem-solving, and skill performance.
- Value flexibility and responsiveness to students' needs and ideas.

Performance Outcomes
- Consider learning objectives when choosing teaching strategies and materials.
- Use strategies to actively engage the learner in critical thinking and problem solving.
- Encourage the student to seek out learning resources outside the classroom.

Criterion Five

The EMS educator understands and utilizes knowledge of individual and group motivation theories and group dynamics to create a positive, engaging learning environment. The following goals will lead toward the accomplishment of this competency.

Cognitive Development
- Understand how to influence group and individual behavior in the educational setting.
- Understand group dynamics.
- Understand the principles and techniques of classroom management and his or her role in maintaining a desirable learning environment.
- Understand barriers to intrinsic motivation.

Affective Development
- Take responsibility for establishing and maintaining a positive, collaborative, engaging learning environment.
- Value the contributions of adult learners to the learning of their peers and colleagues.

Performance Outcomes
- Create an effective adult learning environment.
- Encourage the active engagement of the learner in the educational process.
- Facilitate productive group interaction.
- Establish the behavioral guidelines and policies needed to support an effective learning environment.

Criterion Six

The EMS educator uses knowledge of effective verbal and nonverbal communication and channels of communication to encourage learner inquiry, collaboration, and interaction in the learning environment. To do this he or she should be able to do the following.

Cognitive Development
- Understand cultural and gender influences on the communication process.
- Recognize the importance of both verbal and nonverbal communications.
- Understand the selection of effective media for communication.

Affective Development
- Value the ways in which learners seek to communicate.
- Listen actively and respond thoughtfully to learners.

Performance Outcomes
- Model effective, culturally sensitive verbal and nonverbal communication.
- Use effective techniques of questioning to elicit student responses and encourage discussion.
- Appropriately use educational technology as a means of communication.

Criterion Seven

The EMS educator must be able to competently plan instruction, drawing upon knowledge of subject matter, principles of learning, and goals and objectives of the class or curriculum. In this effort it is necessary to be able to do the following.

Cognitive Development
- Be aware of the process and importance of curriculum development.
- Understand basic principles of learning.
- Be competent in knowledge of subject matter.
- Identify the need to adjust instructional delivery based on student performance.

Affective Development
- Value short-term and long-term planning processes and models in the educational process.
- Be open to evaluation and feedback and their role in ongoing planning.
- Seek the input of colleagues, students, and communities of interest, as appropriate, in the planning process.

Performance Outcomes
- Base plans on the appropriate inputs, processes, and outputs.
- Incorporate knowledge of learning and educational processes into the planning process.
- Respond to unanticipated input.

Criterion Eight

The EMS educator must be able to effectively plan for and utilize both formal and informal techniques of formative and summative evaluation in all facets of the educational program achieving the following.

Cognitive Development
- Understand principles and procedures for classroom and program evaluation.
- Identify appropriate strategies, instruments, and time frames for evaluation of cognitive, affective, and psychomotor achievement.

Affective Development
- Value the processes of student and program evaluation.
- Use assessment to positively direct student development.

Performance Outcomes
- Utilize appropriate, valid measures of student performance.
- Provide feedback to students on the evaluation of their cognitive, affective, and psychomotor development.
- Encourage student self-assessment.
- Analyze the results of assessment.
- Modify instruction as needed on the basis of assessment.
- Maintain useful records of student assessment.

Criterion Nine

The EMS educator is a reflective practitioner who engages in reflection *on* action and reflection *in* action. The EMS educator evaluates and takes responsibility for the impact of his or her decisions and actions and uses self-evaluation to seek opportunities for professional growth. The following are necessary actions in accomplishing this competency.

Cognitive Development
- Be aware of the resources available for self-directed learning.

Affective Development
- Initiate self-assessment.
- Initiate self-directed learning projects for professional development and personal growth.
- Appreciate constructive feedback from students and colleagues.
- Recognize self-assessment and self-directed professional development as professional obligations of the EMS educator.

Performance Outcomes
- Use appropriate means of data collection for self-assessment.
- Seek out valid sources of information and feedback for professional development.

Criterion Ten

The EMS educator cultivates professional relationships with colleagues and stakeholders to improve instruction.

Cognitive Development
- Place the EMS educational program in the context of the EMS community.

Affective Development
- Be an advocate of the learner.
- Cooperate with EMS community stakeholders.

Performance Outcomes
- Participate in activities sponsored by the EMS community.
- Establish relationships with EMS agency educational and administrative personnel.
- Be an advocate of EMS students in the health-care community.

Summary

As an EMS instructor you will assume many roles and carry out responsibilities, or tasks, for those roles. In doing so you will be expected to display the cognitive and affective attributes that are common to all adult educators and those that are more specific to EMS educators. You will need to know the special considerations and terminology for teaching in the traditional classroom, laboratory, and clinical environment. There is much, much more to teaching than simply walking into the classroom and talking about something you know and enjoy. Throughout the rest of this text, you will learn a great deal more about the roles, responsibilities, expectations, and qualities of the EMS educator.

REVIEW QUESTIONS

1. Describe the primary distinction between primary instructors and secondary instructors in EMS.

2. List at least five professional qualities of the adult educator.

3. What are some of the considerations is determining appropriate dress in teaching?

4. What kinds of tasks call for the EMS educator to have effective time-management skills?

5. Provide at least one example of student advocacy.

6. List at least three competencies of the EMS educator.

The Traits
and Needs
of Learners

Learning Objectives

Upon completion of this chapter you should be able to

- Discuss the terms learning style and learning preference.

- Discuss different ways of categorizing learning styles.

- For each learning style presented, suggest teaching methods and learning activities that take advantage of the students' strengths.

- For each learning style presented, propose ways of overcoming the weaknesses associated with it.

- Discuss the impact of personality type on learning styles and preferences.

- Access resources for measuring students' learning styles and preferences.

- Discuss the impact of your own learning style on your teaching.

- Detail the needs and characteristics of adult learners.

- Value individual differences in learning styles and preferences.

- Integrate knowledge of theories of motivation into planning, teaching, evaluation, and counseling activities.

- Discuss how an individual's cultural background influences his or her perceptions and expectations.

- Demonstrate cultural awareness in professional activities.

- Foster cultural awareness among students, faculty, and preceptors.

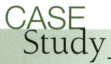

CASE Study

Justin Smith is the primary instructor for an EMT-Intermediate program at St. Mary's Hospital. His class this year is a diverse group, including some volunteer EMTs from a small community about 40 miles away, a couple of college students from the nearby state university campus, some individuals on an industrial emergency response team for their manufacturing company, and several firefighters from the city fire department. Tom Morris, one of the volunteer EMTs, has been with his rescue squad for 15 years and has considerable experience. On the first night of class, two of the firefighters, Andy Boswell and J. T. Long, make it clear that they are in the class only so they can be considered for promotion. One of the individuals from the manufacturing firm, Robert Snowberger, is a retired Army officer and mechanical engineer.

After 3 weeks of class Justin has noticed that Tom Morris seems a little bored with lectures and labs. Andy and J. T are not turning in short assignments or studying for quizzes, and Robert rolls his eyes every time Betsey Whitaker, one of the college students, incorporates a long, drawn-out personal story into a question she asks or an answer she gives.

Questions

1. How could Justin challenge Tom and keep his interest?
2. How might Justin address the fact that Andy and J. T. do not turn in homework?
3. What might be behind Betsey's behavior?
4. Why might Betsey's behavior be especially annoying for Robert?

Introduction

Although there are exceptions, the majority of students with whom you will be interacting are adults or are transitioning to adulthood. As discussed previously, part of the responsibility of an EMS educator is to provide direction needed to students who are in this transition.

Understanding stages of psychosocial and cognitive development makes this task easier. Adults have physical, cognitive, and psychosocial traits that are different from those of less-mature individuals. From your studies in EMS, you already are aware of the physical changes, such as changes in vision and hearing, that occur as we age. You must apply that knowledge to the classroom setting when making decisions, for example, about audiovisual presentations and lighting. In this chapter you will learn about characteristics of adults as learners, theories of motivation, learning styles, and diversity in the classroom. Sensitivity to each of these issues is essential in all your instructional activities, including planning, delivery of instruction, classroom management, counseling, and evaluation.

KEY TERMS

andragogy, p. 80

Bloom's taxonomy of learning, p. 80

concrete operational stage, p. 79

culture, p. 95

epistemology/epistemological, p. 80

extrinsic, p. 89

formal operational stage, p. 79

intrinsic, p. 89

learning style, or preference, p. 85

metacognition, p. 79

motivation, p. 89

neurolinguistic programming, p. 85

postformal stage, p. 80

psychosocial, p. 77

Psychosocial Development

psychosocial
Involving both psychological and social aspects.

Psychosocial development occurs more rapidly during childhood but continues across the life span. Levinson and Levinson (1996) propose that psychosocial development takes place in a predictable, chronological order. Their theory is that we go through sequential periods of psychosocial stability and transition. These time periods are shown in Box 6-1.

Erik Erikson's theory of psychosocial development is sequential, but beyond childhood it does not tie each stage to an exact chronological age. Each of his stages represents two alternative developmental paths, one positive and one negative. Adolescents struggle with identity versus identity confusion. It is in this stage that adolescents try alternative approaches to their behavior in order to make identity-congruent decisions as adults regarding career, marriage, and other life decisions. The

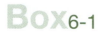

Box6-1

Levinson and Levinson's Sequential Theory of Adult Psychosocial Development
(Levinson and Levinson 1996, 18)

Early Adult Transition	*Ages 17–22*
Entry-life structure for early adulthood	Ages 22–28
Age 30 Transition	*Ages 28–33*
Culminating structure for early adulthood	Ages 33–40
Midlife Transition	*Ages 40–45*
Early-life structure for middle adulthood	Ages 45–50
Age 50 Transition	*Ages 50–55*
Culminating life structure for middle adulthood	Ages 55–60
Late Adult Transition	*Ages 60–65*
Late adulthood	Age 60 and beyond

struggles to become independent from parents and to form an identity are somewhat isolating. As we enter young adulthood we struggle with intimacy and finding love versus isolation. During young adulthood the task is to develop the ability to care for and share with others. Middle-aged adults struggle with generativity versus self-absorption. During this stage, the struggle is between the individual productivity expected in western society and the ability to care for others, such as children and aging parents. Older adults struggle with integrality versus despair. At this stage adults either come to terms with the life choices they have made and feel a sense of satisfaction or become bitter because of lost opportunities. Some theorists believe that these conflicts can recur at times during life. For example, the death of a spouse or divorce may cause the intimacy versus isolation conflict to arise again. Awareness of developmental theories will help give you an understanding of the behaviors, interests, motivations, and distractions of your students.

PEARLS *Often people are engaged in the struggles of two stages at once and are rarely in only one stage at a given time.*

Cognitive and Moral Development

There are a number of theories of cognitive and moral development. Much of the research done on cognitive and moral development has been in children. Theories about adult cognitive and moral development are still emerging. The primary focus here is cognitive development. For a discussion on adult moral development, refer to Chapter 3. The primary criticisms of Jean Piaget's stages of cognitive development (Box 6-2) are that they imply that cognitive development is complete in early adolescence and that the same course of development applies to all individuals. In fact, a significant number of adults never reach the formal operational stage of thinking—a situation you will recognize when a student struggles with understanding that, for example, even though asthmatics wheeze, not all wheezing in the lungs is caused by asthma or that it is not necessary to immobilize every patient from a motor vehicle collision on a long backboard. Additionally, it has been proposed that there are stages of cognitive development beyond the formal operational stage.

Piaget proposed that children reach the **concrete operational stage** of thinking at about age 6 and the **formal operational stage** of cognitive development around the age of 11. Concrete operational thinking is characterized by an either-or orientation and by a lack of tolerance for ambiguity. At this stage it is assumed that there is a widely applicable "right" answer to all situations and that there is an inability to consider multiple variables in a situation. Formal operational thinking is characterized by hypothetical thinking and deductive reasoning, as well as **metacognition,** or the ability to think about one's own thinking and learning processes. However, the limitations to formal operational thinking are that it is purely logical and does not involve the affective domain, it focuses on finding solutions to problems that are presented but does not allow for recognition problems (problem finding), and it uses a single system of reference.

concrete operational stage
A phase of cognitive development occurring at about 6 years of age. The ability to think abstractly is not well developed.

formal operational stage
A stage of cognitive development that begins at about 11 years of age. Transition to this stage is marked by the capacity for abstract thought.

metacognition
The ability to think about one's own thinking processes.

Box 6-2

Piaget's Stages of Cognitive Development

Birth to age 2 years	Sensoriomotor
2 to 6 years	Preoperational
6 to 11 years	Concrete operational
11 years through adulthood	Formal operational

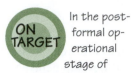

In the postformal operational stage of cognitive development, individuals are able to consider the context of problems and solve problems with multiple variables and no clear answers.

Other theorists have proposed that there is a **postformal stage** of thinking in which the individual considers the contextual relevance of situations. The essential hallmark of postformal thinking is the ability to deal with multivariate tasks that do not have a universally accepted answer. This involves the levels of cognitive functioning described in **Bloom's taxonomy of learning** (about which you will learn more later in the text) as analysis, synthesis, and evaluation.

Other theories of cognitive development differentiate cognitive styles not only by level, but by gender as well. Marcia Baxter Magolda's **epistemological** reflection model (Severiens, Dam, and Nijenhuis 1998) proposes four levels of learning, three of which show gender-related differences in patterns of reasoning. Epistemology refers to different ways of knowing, or of constructing knowledge. The Epistemological Reflection Model is summarized in Box 6-3.

Andragogy

postformal stage
A stage of cognitive development occurring beyond adolescence characterized by the ability not only to solve, but also to recognize problems.

Bloom's taxonomy of learning
A systematic, hierarchical classification of types and levels of learning.

epistemology/ epistemological
A theory of the nature of knowledge.

andragogy
The teaching of adults, as opposed to pedagogy, the teaching of children.

Andragogy is a theory of adult learning that is most often associated with Malcolm Knowles. Although he did not coin the term, he did develop the theory and popularize the term. For clarification, there are some educational experts who consider andragogy not to be a theory, but more a set of assumptions about adult learners and effective methods of adult education. In the past, some texts have promoted andragogy as the only theory of adult education, although there are many theories and models. It is useful to discuss andragogy here, because it addresses some common traits and needs of adult learners. Malcolm Knowles (1980) put forward six assumptions about adult learners, each of which provides insight into the expectations and behaviors of adults in learning situations. It is important to remember that these are broad generalizations and that the needs and characteristics underlying these assumptions may not be manifest in all adult learners. Human beings are complex, and understanding them and their motivations for learning cannot be reduced to six simple assumptions. Nonetheless, you and your students will benefit from your familiarity with these ideas.

Assumption 1: Adults Need to Know Why They Need to Learn Something

The first assumption, that adults need to know why they need to learn something, points to the importance of explaining the relevance of a lesson to the learner's goals and needs. Often these needs and goals can be as general as the need to do a good a job and to be perceived as competent

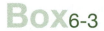

Box 6-3

The Epistemological Reflection Model of Cognitive Development Stages
(Severiens, Dam, and Nijenhuis 1998)

ABSOLUTE KNOWING

Teachers are seen as the absolute authority on subject matter and learning material consists of absolute truths. Teachers are supposed to supply the answers and learners at this level want to demonstrate learning of "the facts."

Receiving pattern: Seen more frequently in women than men. Students tend to listen passively to the teacher to receive knowledge.

Mastering pattern: More often seen in men. Students in the mastering pattern ask more questions, challenge the teacher, and look for points of argumentation. Expect the teacher to be entertaining and want to interact with peers.

TRANSITIONAL KNOWING

The student realizes that authorities do not know everything there is to know about a subject. Wants to apply knowledge, not just demonstrate learning of facts

Interpersonal pattern: More often seen in women. There is a trust that all beliefs are equally true and that tests should incorporate individual differences. Wants to hear the beliefs and opinions of peers.

Impersonal pattern: Seen more often in men. The student is directed toward certainty and problem solving. The student believes that uncertainty can be resolved by authorities, logic, or research.

INDEPENDENT KNOWING

The student is concerned with creating his/her own perspective and believes that the teacher should promote independent thought. The belief is that tests should reward the ability to think and reason independently.

Interindividual pattern: More often women than men. Belief that knowledge is uncertain because everyone constructs knowledge differently and that personal experience plays a significant role in knowledge.

Individual pattern: More often men than women. Consider their own perspectives first and have difficulty listening to other perspectives. Prefers to set own learning goals. Belief that everyone has a point of view, but that one's own point of view should be maintained.

CONTEXTUAL KNOWING

Belief that knowledge is uncertain, but that not every idea is equally valid. Validity of knowledge is based on evidence supporting the knowledge. This stage is reached by the least number of adults and the model was unable to detect patterns in reasoning because of the small numbers.

---

in one's job. Other times, you will find yourself explaining how today's lesson is related to next week's lesson, for which the need may be more obvious. Yet, other adults have a lifelong learning orientation and enjoy learning for learning's sake.

Assumption 2: Adults Have a Deep Need to Be Seen by Others as Being Self-Directing

The self-directing nature of adults underscores the importance of providing choices and latitude in the means of accomplishing objectives, to the extent possible within the regulatory framework of EMS education. As a simple example of respecting self-direction, it is not appropriate to have adults raise their hands to ask permission to use the restroom during class. Although it is common practice to require that students explain the reasons for absences, you should carefully consider whether this is congruent with the self-directing nature of adults. If we believe that adults are self-directing, then we must believe that they are making decisions based on the priorities of a mature person and with full awareness of the consequences of their decisions. To question adults' decisions about their life priorities is to question their ability to be self-directing. You may experience adult students' resentment of the implication that you are asking to judge the validity of their absence.

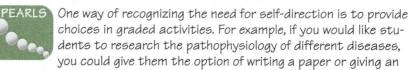

Assumption 3: Adults Have a Greater Quantity and Different Quality of Experience

That adults come into educational situations with more experiences is both helpful and obstructive to learning. Prior experience can serve as a framework to which new concepts can be connected. It is, in fact, very important to appeal to adults' experiences in the teaching-learning transaction. This is the very nature of progressive education—learning progresses through the continuity of prior experiences with current and future experiences. However, when prior experience is—or at least seems to the learner to be—contrary to the material being presented, it is an obstacle to learning. For example, each time there is a change in CPR or ACLS, it is very difficult for people who have learned one way to begin doing it the new way. This is especially true because such courses focus on rote memorization of material and mechanization of skills, rather than on problem solving and critical thinking. In a similar vein, there have been First Responder and EMT students who found it difficult to believe that applying butter or bacon grease to burns is not in the patient's best interest, because this was the home treatment that their families had used successfully, in their experience, for generations. It is essential to proceed with caution is such instances. Adults define themselves through their experiences. Any attempt or perceived attempt to contradict this experience can be a threat to the ego or can be perceived as disrespectful of the original source of the information. However, we are obligated to correct incorrect information insofar as it is related to the content of the course.

Assumption 4: Adults Are Ready to Learn Things That Can Immediately Help Them Cope with a Life Need

Although this may be true, it does not mean that adults seek learning *only* to satisfy an immediate need. The need may be at a higher, less-tangible level and not so immediate, as you will come to see when you read about motivation theories. Other theorists promote the concept that many adults have an orientation toward lifelong learning.

Assumption 5: Adults Are Problem-Centered Learners, Versus Subject-Centered Learners

Problem-centered learning is appealing to younger and adult learners alike. It is not that children do not prefer problem-centered learning, it is just that they are traditionally taught in a subject-based curriculum. Although it is necessary to supply subject matter to the degree necessary to provide students with an adequate foundation for problem solving, most students enjoy lab and clinical rotations tremendously because of their problem-based orientation. One way to establish the "why" of the lesson is to begin with a scenario or case study that the students can't solve with existing knowledge. This stimulates an interest in the information needed to solve the problem.

Assumption 6: Adults' Motivations to Learn Are Intrinsic

Often children are motivated to demonstrate learning to please a teacher or a parent. This is because the learning that takes place in the formal school curriculum is not the students' choice of learning activities. Because there is not a free choice in learning activities, schools rely on *extrinsic* rewards to elicit the desired behavior. This is not the case with the adult learner. As discussed previously, we can help adults see how the educational program can meet a need or perhaps remove barriers to motivation, but we cannot provide the motivation. For example, if the student enters the program without sufficient awareness of what an EMS provider does, an explanation of the scope of practice may be appealing to the learner, who may then be motivated to learn the material needed to carry out the roles and responsibilities of an EMS provider. In this case, you have helped remove a barrier to motivation by providing information. If the adult student is attending a class by mandate against his or her wishes, the motivation will be to do what is necessary to get out of an unpleasant situation or to avoid the punishment (formal disciplinary action, lack of promotion, unappealing job assignments) associated with course failure.

Learning Styles and Preferences

learning style, or preference
The particular way that an individual prefers to take in and process information.

neurolinguistic programming
A classification of learning styles based on the sensory modality by which one prefers to take in information.

Learning styles are multidimensional. The term **learning style**, or **preference,** refers to what people select to concentrate on, how they concentrate on particular stimuli, and how they process information and make meaning of it to learn new information and skills. There are many different ways of looking at learning styles and preferences. Some are more global and try to assess all the dimensions related to learning, whereas others are more focused on selected dimensions of learning. Some of the more well-known learning style theories are those of Dunn and Dunn, Kolb, Honey and Mumford, and Gardner (Merriam and Caffarella 2000). There are also hemispheric dominance theories that focus on right- or left-brain dominance and **neurolinguistic programming** models. These theories and models are not contradictory but, instead, focus on different processes or aspects of learning. As with all theories and models, they have their strengths and limitations, and as you read more about them beyond the scope of this book, you will find that each has its critics and supporters.

It is important to point out that, although we may have preferences for the way we learn and we may be more comfortable and successful learning in particular ways, we can all learn in a variety of ways. It is equally important to point out that a learner's preferences are not necessarily his or her strengths. Still another important concept is that we tend to teach as we learn. That is, our preferred way of teaching is linked to our preferred way of learning. As you learn more about your own learning style, you will come to understand why you prefer some teaching strategies and activities to others. (*Author's note:* From insight into my own cognitive style, I know that the reason I prefer not to be a practical-exam evaluator is that I'm impatient with details and dislike doing the same thing over and over.) Nonetheless, as an educator you will need to learn to become comfortable with teaching in a variety of ways.

There is a wide assortment of instruments that can help identify learning styles. Some of these are freely available, whereas others must be purchased and/or administered by someone specially qualified to interpret the results and counsel the student regarding the use of the results. With some knowledge of some of the theories of learning styles and some astute observation, you will develop the ability to make educated guesses about your students' learning styles. With knowledge of students' learning styles, you will be able to provide suggestions to students for activities to enhance learning. All of this may leave you wondering how you are to meet all these different needs. As a rule, teach the class as a whole first, using a variety of techniques. You cannot adapt your teaching style to meet the needs of only a few students in the class, but by providing activities that appeal to all learners at one time or another, you will keep students' interest. Requiring students to learn by various methods also helps them to grow and to increase their capacity for learning.

Dunn and Dunn's Learning-Style Inventory

The Dunn and Dunn instrument assesses the learner's reaction to 23 different elements in five dimensions, or strands, of learning. These five strands are environmental, emotional, social, physiological, and psychological. The environmental strand includes preferences for the amount or type of lighting in the learning environment, whether or not sound, such as music or television in the background, is favored over complete silence, the temperature of the environment, and whether or not a formal or informal seating arrangement is preferred. Emotional aspects include motivation, persistence, and the need for internal or external structure of learning. The social dimension includes preferences for learning alone, with a peer or mentor, in small groups, or as a team. Physiological preferences are based on preferred sensory stimulation, needs for food or drink while studying, peak times of day for energy, and whether or not one needs to be able to move about in the environment.

Kolb's Experiential Learning Styles

David Kolb's theory of learning styles represents four learning styles that are the product of the interaction of a vertical axis representing a spectrum from abstract conceptualization (thinking) to concrete experience (feeling) and a horizontal axis representing a continuum from active experimentation (doing) to reflective observation (watching) (Jones, Reichard, and Mokhtari 2003). See Figure 6-1. Each of the quadrants formed by

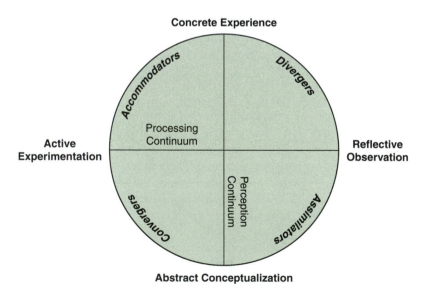

Figure 6-1
Kolb's Learning Styles
Adapted from Jones, Reichard, and Mokhtari (2003).

these axes represents a different learning style, which reflects differences in perceiving and processing information. Those who use a combination of doing and feeling are called accommodators. Those who use a combination of feeling and watching are called divergers. People who use a combination of watching and thinking are known as assimilators, and those who use a combination of thinking and doing are called convergers. This is a popular model, and a search on the Internet will lead you to multiple sites for additional information, many of which are constructed by schools of education in major universities.

Honey and Mumford's Theory of Learning Styles

Honey and Mumford, whose theory is influenced by Kolb, describe four types of learners: activists, reflectors, theorists, and pragmatists (Carney 2000). Activists focus on the here and now and enjoy new experiences but become bored with repetition. They respond well to hands-on activities. Reflectors like to view and evaluate situations from different vantage points. They learn well from watching others and asking them questions. Theorists like to think problems through logically, sequentially, and systematically and are easily able to assimilate isolated concepts into a cohesive theory. Pragmatists enjoy the opportunity to quickly apply theories to practice and benefit from classroom learning followed by laboratory or clinical experiences.

Neurolinguistic Programming

Neurolinguistic programming focuses on the preferred sensory modality of receiving information. Some people prefer auditory stimulation and like to receive information from listening to others. They benefit from tape-recording lectures and engaging in discussion. Other people pay attention to and more easily take in visual stimuli and benefit from pictures, diagrams, observations, and models. Still other individuals are kinesthetic (sometimes called tactile) learners and prefer to learn by doing. It is sometimes possible to listen for clues to the auditory, visual, and kinesthetic (AVK) preferences in dialogues with students. For example, the visual learner may respond to you by saying, "I see what you mean by that." The auditory learner may say something such as, "I hear what you are saying." The kinesthetic learner may say something like, "I can't quite put my finger on what bothers me about that." A variation of AVK is VARK™, which includes reading in addition to visual, auditory, and kinesthetic preferences. You can learn more about and take the VARK™ inventory at **http://www.vark-learn.com/english/page.asp?p=advice**.

Multiple Intelligences

Howard Gardner's (1983) theory of multiple intelligences is a bit different in that it proposes that there are not just preferred ways of learning, but that intelligence takes many forms. Gardner identifies eight different kinds of intelligence. Linguistic/verbal intelligence is the ability to learn from and convey thoughts through language. Such people are usually good at determining the nuances between similar concepts and explaining concepts to others. Musical intelligence, because of its symbolic (i.e., linguistic) nature and because of its rhythmic, metric nature, is related to both verbal/linguistic and mathematical/logical intelligences. Mathematical/logical intelligence refers to the ability to detect patterns, sequences, and relationships. Spatial intelligence refers to the ability to perceive physical relationships of objects, such as would be important in, for example, driving. Bodily/kinesthetic intelligence is the ability to easily learn and perform complex coordinated physical tasks. Interpersonal intelligence refers to the ability to perceive and understand the emotions and motivations of other people, as is important in being empathetic. Intrapersonal intelligence is the ability to know and have insight about one's self. Environmental, or naturalist, intelligence refers to the ability to appreciate and interact with the natural environment and understand the natural order of things in the environment.

PEARLS Gardner's theory can be used to explain differences between students when it comes to "people skills," classroom learning, and laboratory learning.

General Resources for Information about Learning Styles

The preceding discussion does not address all learning-styles theories, nor does it talk about the theories extensively. The following websites provide additional information about the learning-styles theories discussed here and others as well.

- http://www.learning-styles-online.com/overview/
- http://fcis.oise.utoronto.ca/~daniel_schugurensky/faqs/qa20.html
- http://www.clat.psu.edu/gems/Other/LSI/LSI.htm
- http://www.indstate.edu/ctl/styles/ls1.html
- http://www.oswego.edu/CandI/plsi/
- http://www.nwlink.com/~donclark/hrd/learning/styles.html

Influence of Personality

Some of the learning style theories discussed here are based on the personality theory developed by Carl Jung. The Myers-Briggs type indicator (MBTI) is also based on Jungian theory. Not only can it be applied to learning, but it also applies to other elements of cognitive and psychosocial functioning as well. One of the ways our personalities are expressed is through our mental habits, which are identified by the MBTI. Our "types" influence what we pay attention to, what is important to us, and how we make decisions. There are 16 different types identified by the MBTI. Each is a combination of four letters that stands for opposed preferences on four dimensions. The four dimensions and their characteristics are summarized in Box 6-4. It is important that the MBTI, as with all such instruments for measuring personality and learning styles, is used not to stereotype or categorize people, but to understand behavioral tendencies. All such instruments are somewhat reductionistic, because there is not a single instrument that can address the complexity of human personality. Because of the complexity of interpreting the nuances of the MBTI, it is administered only by personnel who are certified by the Center for Applications of Psychological Type (CAPT). There may be someone in the student services or human resources development department of your institution who is qualified to administer the MBTI.

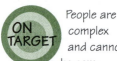 *People are complex and cannot be completely explained by a battery of tests and instruments to measure personality and learning styles.*

Theories of Motivation

motivation
An internal drive to meet an unmet need.

Motivation can be defined as "the set of processes that arouse, direct, and maintain human behavior toward attaining some goal" (Baron and Greenberg 2000, 130). Most definitions of motivation relate arousal to the presence of an unmet need. This is easy to comprehend if we consider that when all our needs are satisfied, at least for the moment, we are not motivated toward activity. An unmet need serves as the drive behind behavior, yet we make choices about how we will go about satisfying that need. These choices about how we will attempt to meet our needs constitute the direction of our behavior. The maintenance of goal-directed behavior is determined by the level of persistence a person has for meeting a goal. Persistence is related to the perceived importance of the goal and the belief that one's continued actions will result in attaining that goal. By thinking of motivation as a drive to meet an unmet need, it is clear that motivation is **intrinsic.** That is, it comes from within the person, because the unmet need is internal to the person and can be experienced only by that person. Even so-called **extrinsic** motivators must appeal to

intrinsic
Originating from within an individual.

extrinsic
Originating from outside an individual.

Box6-4

Dimensions of the MBTI
(Lawrence 1993).

EXTROVERSION (E)—INTROVERSION (I)

E: Likes action and variety, likes to see how other people perform tasks, thinks and solves problems "out loud" by talking to others, wants to know what other people expect of him or her.

I: Likes to have quiet and time for contemplation, thinks things through before speaking, needs to understand the principles and ideas behind a task, prefers to work alone.

SENSING (S)–INTUITION (N)

S: Takes experiences at face value, uses the senses to find out what is going on around him or her, good at memorizing facts and details, but impatient when details are complicated, prefers to solve problems with which there is prior experience.

N: Pays attention to the "big picture," uses imagination and sees possibilities, dislikes repetition, enjoys solving new problems, but impatient with details.

THINKING (T)–FEELING (F)

T: May overlook others' feelings or hurt their feelings without realizing it, pays more attention to ideas than people, values logic and a sense of justice and fair play, does not need harmony to function in a group.

F: Makes decisions based on personal values, likes to be praised, is aware of and can predict others' feelings, disturbed by disharmony in a group.

JUDGING (J)–PERCEIVING (P)

J: Likes to have a plan and stick to it, has a notion of how things "ought" to be, likes to finish one project before starting another, wants to be right, may decide before getting all the details, adheres to schedules and standards that are not easy to adjust.

P: Likes to keep options open and be flexible, deals easily with the unexpected, makes changes "on the fly," starts many projects but has trouble following through, may delay decisions while seeking more information.

---

some unmet need of the person—whether it is for money or recognition or some other need. For example, even though grades are considered external motivators, a student will not work for a grade unless the grade is important to him or her. In this section you will learn about theories of motivation and how they apply to the educational setting.

Maslow's Hierarchy of Needs

One of the most well-known theories of motivation is Maslow's hierarchy of needs. Abraham Maslow contended that human beings have five types of needs, grouped in two categories, and that these needs are activated successively from more basic, lower-level needs to higher-order needs. The deficiency needs are categorized as physiological needs, safety needs, and social needs, whereas the growth needs are for esteem and self-actualization.

The most basic needs are at the physiological level. These needs are related to survival and include such things as having food, water, and shelter. Higher-order needs are not activated until survival needs are satisfied, at least to some degree. This need to provide the necessities of life explains why people will tolerate a less-than-ideal work situation that does not meet higher-order needs, if their only choices are to stay with the job and be able to survive or leave the job and face the possibility of hunger and homelessness. Providing breaks during class time allows students to meet their needs for food, drink, rest, and physical activity. By providing these breaks and allowing for the satisfaction of basic needs, you will allow the opportunity for students' higher-order needs to be activated.

Safety needs include both physical and psychological freedom from threat and harm. On the job, this can include the provision of safety gear and workplace policies, such as tenure, that provide for safety and security. In the learning environment the student must feel free to ask questions without the threat of ridicule by the instructor or classmates. Students must also know that they can express their concerns without fear of retribution.

People also have social needs, which are activated after satisfactory fulfillment of physiological and safety needs. Social needs include people's desires to have friends, to be accepted, and to participate in social activities. Educational settings provide opportunities to meet others with the same interests. You will often notice how relationships form in a class and how the class becomes a community, rather than a collection of disconnected individuals. You may also notice that close to break times, there tends to more chatting among the students. Giving adequate breaks, as well as building in interactive class activities, allows people's social needs to be satisfied.

According to Maslow, if these three lower-level needs are not met, there will be physical harm or illness and psychological maladjustment, such that a person's functioning is diminished. The two higher needs, esteem and self-actualization, are known as growth needs and function to allow individuals to reach their fullest potential.

Esteem needs are people's needs to have self-respect and the approval of others. Self-esteem may suffer at work when, for example, employer policies restrict taking actions in the best interests of others, creating an ethical and moral dilemma for employees. They may feel forced to act in a manner that lowers their self-respect in order to meet the more basic need of maintaining employment. In the classroom, the need for approval can be addressed through sincere praise and expression of appreciation for contributions.

The need for self-actualization is activated after other needs are sufficiently satisfied. A student's purpose for taking your class may be a step toward his or her self-actualization, just as taking an instructor course and participating in lifelong learning may be a step toward your own self-actualization. It is generally thought that very few people become completely self-actualized, but that the need to be self-actualized is what keeps us motivated to grow and develop throughout life.

Alderfer's ERG Theory

Alderfer's ERG theory is similar to Maslow's hierarchy of needs, but it expresses needs more generally as the needs for existence, relatedness, and growth. Existence is related to Maslow's physiological and safety needs, relatedness corresponds to Maslow's social needs, and growth is related to Maslow's esteem and self-actualization needs.

Goal-setting Theories

Goal-setting theories are premised on the ideas that people need to feel competent in what they are doing and that dissatisfaction occurs when there is a discrepancy between actual performance and a clear goal. Locke and Latham (Baron and Greenberg 2000) propose that motivation occurs when a person is committed to a goal and believes in his or her ability to attain that goal. It is important to realize that the motivation is still intrinsic, even though the goal may have been set by someone else. If the student is not committed to the goal and/or does not believe that his or her efforts will result in attaining the goal, he or she will not be motivated. If you choose to use goal setting as an instructor, you must make sure that the goals are specific and challenging—but attainable. Additionally, it is important to provide feedback on the progress toward the goal so that the student realizes his or her efforts are making a difference. Finally, it is important to involve students in the goal-setting process to ensure that the goal is important to the student and thereby enhance student commitment to the goal.

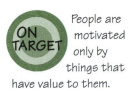 People are motivated only by things that have value to them.

Justice Theories

Equity theory suggests that there is a social component to motivation in that individuals are motivated to maintain equitable, or fair, relationships with others. Students tend to compare their outputs and rewards to others and to the program standards. Equitability refers to the social comparison of one's self against others. In the classroom, a student may feel that he or she put as much or more effort into a paper or studying for an exam than a classmate did. If the classmate receives a better grade, the first student may become angry. In this case, anger is the intrinsic stimulus for which the student seeks satisfaction. The student's behavior in this case is often to challenge the instructor about his or her grade for the assignment or exam. Although we must always be humble enough to consider our grading practices and the validity of assignments and exams, often the challenge is to help the student see that, even though his or her efforts are commendable, we must grade on outcomes, for this is what matters in EMS practice. One way to forestall such an incident is to set a climate of peer cooperation, rather than competition. This is sometimes difficult though, because of the individualistic orientation of people in the United States.

The preceding example relates to distributive justice, or how rewards are distributed within a group. Procedural justice refers to the perceived fairness of the decision-making processes. Perceived procedural justice can be increased by allowing students to have a say in decision making, admitting and correcting errors in decision making, being consistent in the application of policies, and remaining unbiased in decision making. It is important to treat students with respect and maintain their dignity during decision-making processes, too.

Expectancy Theory

Expectancy theory is based on the concepts of expectancy, instrumentality, and valence. Expectancy is the belief that one's efforts will result in desired outputs. For example, a student will not be motivated to study if he or she has poor study skills and studying has not resulted in satisfactory academic performance in the past.

Instrumentality refers to the belief that efforts and their associated outputs will lead to a reward. This is an argument for criterion-referenced grading versus norm-referenced grading (which you will learn more about when you read on the subject of student assessment). In criterion-referenced grading, student performance is measured against a standard, and all students stand an equal chance of getting, say, a grade of A. Norm-referenced grading refers to "grading on a curve," which puts students in competition with each other. In this case a student who would otherwise have gotten a B might get a lower grade, depending on the performance of other students, even though his or her performance was high.

The valence of a reward refers to its meaning or significance to the student. Even if a student believes that hard work will result in output and will be rewarded, less effort may be expended if the reward means little to the student. In this situation it is easy to see why a student trying to get into medical school highly values the contribution of a grade of A to his or her overall grade-point average (GPA), whereas a student who is not taking the course for credit may care little about a grade of A. It is important to remember that other motivational factors may come into play as well. The non-credit-seeking student may not care about the A but may care very much about being competent, regardless of the grade.

Effects of Culture and Gender

As you read earlier in the chapter, there appear to be some differences between males and females in terms of cognitive styles at different levels of cognitive development. Currently there is evidence that not only are males and females socialized differently, but there also may be biological differences in male and female brains that explain these differences. In general, women tend to think of things contextually and with regard to relationships, whereas men tend to view knowledge as logical and absolute. Regardless of the underlying causes, one way of perceiving and processing information and relating to the world is not inferior to the other. It is important to remember that the differences are true in general only and that each individual is unique and must not be stereotyped by these differences.

There are cultural differences of which you should be aware, too. Depending on where you live in North America, there are varying degrees of cultural diversity. In fact, a number of estimates put minority populations at more than one-third of the total population. This number is expected to keep increasing in years to come. Your background may be rich with experiences with other cultures, or you may have been brought up in and lived in a culturally homogenous area. Increasingly, there are opportunities for involvement in international EMS education projects that can also give you opportunities to interact with people from different cultures. It is beyond the scope of this book to discuss cultural differences in depth. The primary focus here is to present some of the areas in which there are different cultural expectations. It is up to you to become culturally competent in your particular environment. You can find a wealth of information on the topic at **http://www. diversityhotwire.com/index.php**.

culture
Socially transmitted behavior patterns, beliefs, and values.

Culture is the behavioral expression of social and religious customs and the aesthetic and intellectual norms of a group of people. People have cultural differences as to whom one is to show respect and how respect is demonstrated, in beliefs about men's and women's roles, modesty, participation in childbirth, and care of patients by members of the opposite sex, and in preferences for personal space and touching. Even when a nonnative English-speaking student is proficient in the English language, there are nuances of meaning in the use of words and body language that may cause miscommunication. Additionally, there are cultural differences in giving and receiving feedback in the educational setting. Consider the following scenarios.

Scenario 1

A student in your EMT-B class, Jae Lin, seems to be having difficulty understanding the concept of shock. In response to her seemingly puzzled expression, you ask if she understands the material. She says yes, and you continue on. This situation repeats itself several times over the next couple of lectures. Upon grading exams, you find it apparent that Jae Lin didn't have an adequate understanding of concepts. Unbeknownst to you, when Jae Lin was saying yes, she meant that she was listening politely to you, not that she understood the material.

Scenario 2

You are teaching a class of 20 Iranian men who are taking a paramedic course. In making clinical assignments, you find that they are extremely uncomfortable with and object to the idea of observing, let alone participating in, childbirth. How could you approach the situation?

Scenario 3

You have students from Norway, Japan, Greece, and Brazil in your EMT-B class. Do you think any of these students will be more comfortable than others in touching or being touched by other students in patient-assessment lab?

Scenario 4

Tran is one of your advisees and comes to talk to you about his frustration with one of his instructors. He says," Karen always tells me my English is good. My English is not good. She is my teacher; she should not tell me my English is good when it isn't. She should tell me to work harder and be better."

Unfortunately, when we are not comfortable with other cultures, we tend to ignore, rather than explore, differences. Even well-educated Americans tend to know little about other cultures. Be careful not to stereotype and make assumptions based on biological similarities or nationality (*Author's note:* I once heard a doctoral-level classmate ask an Indian [Hindi] student if she was fasting for Ramadan, a Muslim holy tradition). Find out as much as you can about other cultures by speaking informally with people. Because EMS is a helping profession, not only must you as the instructor be culturally aware, but also you must strive to create an atmosphere of cultural understanding in the classroom. There are a number of ways you can accomplish this. Some suggestions are provided in Box 6-5.

Box 6-5

Suggestions for Increasing Cultural Awareness in the Classroom

- Start class discussions by asking about holidays and how special events such as births and weddings are celebrated.
- For the first several classes, have one or two students per class session bring in one or two "personal artifacts," such as photographs, mementos, etc., to show and talk about.
- When discussing therapeutic communications, ask about the meaning of different nonverbal gestures cross-culturally.
- When teaching about death and grief, ask about the customs of other countries and cultures.
- Ask about home and folk remedies, alternative medicine, and cultural beliefs about illness.
- When talking about life-span development, offer the opportunity to talk about the roles of different family members.
- When talking about geriatrics, ask about the differences in how the elderly are perceived and treated in different cultures.

Summary

The focus of this chapter has been on understanding human behavior. You should be completing this chapter with a sense of how learning styles, levels of cognitive, psychosocial, and moral development, motivation, personality, culture, and gender affect human learning and behavior. Knowledge of these topics allows you to better understand the processes behind behavior, how to help students understand themselves better, and how to be an effective instructor for a wide variety of individuals with differing needs and preferences.

REVIEW QUESTIONS

1. According to Erik Erikson's theory of psychosocial development, at about what age in life are individuals likely to be struggling with a need to be productively involved in their work and a need to care for older and younger generations?

2. What are the characteristics of concrete operational thinking?

3. What are the six assumptions of andragogy?

4. How might Howard Gardner's multiple-intelligences theory help you explain differences in student learning?

5. What theory of motivation explains decreased effort when the effort is not perceived as likely to change the outcome for the individual?

6. List two activities you could use to promote cultural awareness in a diverse classroom.

The Psychology of Learning

Learning Objectives

Upon completion of this chapter you should be able to

- Define learning.

- Discuss the concepts of progressivism and constructivism as they relate to learning.

- Explain the roles of working memory and long-term memory in learning.

- Relate the role of experience to learning.

- Describe the importance of reflection on experience.

- Explain the usefulness and limitations of models of the learning process.

- Describe the three domains of learning.

- Provide examples of activities within each domain of learning.

CASE Study _____

Danielle LaFollette is getting ready to prepare a lesson plan for teaching airway management in her EMT-Basic course. Because she is a new instructor, it seems like an overwhelming task. Danielle is conscientious and wants to make sure that her lesson plan not only contains the right information, but that the sequence and methods she uses are effective in facilitating students' learning. She wants students to appreciate the importance of airway management, understand the consequences of poor airway management, and to be skilled in providing airway management.

Questions

1. What would be an effective way for Danielle to sequence the material?
2. How can Danielle make the presentation of material most effective?
3. In which domains of learning should Danielle be writing objectives?

Introduction

In this chapter we learn about the process of learning from neurobiological and psychological perspectives. We discuss the brain, memory, and cognitive structures, as well as theories and models of the learning process. Finally, we discuss the cognitive, affective, and psychomotor domains of learning, and the types of actions that correspond to each category. Before you begin reading this material, you will need to have a working understanding of the term *learning*. At its most basic level, learning is defined as a relatively permanent change in behavior that takes place as a result of experience. The behavior may be cognitive, in terms of changes in perspective and ways of thinking; or it may be affective: a change in attitudes or values. Learning bodily or using kinesthetic skills is known as psychomotor learning. Different types of experiences have varying levels of value in learning. For example, hearing someone describe the care of a trauma patient is not as powerful as actually being a part of the situation and seeing, touching, and hearing the patient and the things going on around him. Additionally, John Dewey (1938) describes experiences as educative only if they connect with other experiences and lead to growth. Growth and continuity of experience are the two factors used to judge the educational value of an experience. A miseducative experience occurs when the result is to limit or narrow further experience and growth. Growth from experience occurs due to reflection on the experience and is expressed when it changes the nature of a subsequent experience. This is what we mean by the **transfer of learning.**

transfer of learning The use of knowledge or skills learned in one situation or environment in a new situation or environment.

KEY TERMS

affective domain, p. 110

cognitive domain, p. 110

constructivism, p. 105

echoic memory, p. 103

experiential learning, p. 108

extrinsic cognitive load, p. 105

iconic memory, p. 103

Psychological and Neurobiological Processes in Learning

The psychological or mental process of learning is referred to as cognition, or cognitive ability. The study of cognition is concerned with how we select, receive, process, store, use, and convey knowledge. Neurobiology is concerned with the structural, chemical, and electrical mechanisms of the brain. The best way to understand the process of learning is to consider both aspects together.

Neurobiological Considerations

Much of what we know about the brain and its functioning comes from animal studies and observations of patients with traumatic brain injury, stroke, or other organic brain lesions. The advent of diagnostic imaging techniques, such as magnetic resonance imaging and positron emission tomography, has allowed for additional insight into the functions of the brain.

The cerebral hemispheres of the brain are connected by and communicate with each other via the corpus callosum, a neurofibrous bundle. The right and left hemispheres differ to some degree in their functioning. The left brain processes logical, analytical, and mathematical types of information, whereas the right brain processes artistic, musical, and emotional information. The fact that the hemispheres communicate with each other allows us to integrate complex information, such as the content of conversation (left brain) and the quality and pitch of the voices (right brain). The cerebral hemispheres contain the limbic system, which arose earlier in evolution, and the neocortex, a later evolutionary feature. The neocortex is divided into the frontal, temporal, parietal, and occipital lobes of the brain.

Memory and emotion are associated in the brain and not separate from each other. You have most likely experienced the memories and emotions associated with an aroma from earlier experiences or from a song that played a prominent role in earlier experiences. The structures of the limbic system, including the amygdala, thalamus, hypothalamus, and hippocampus, function to process emotions and memories, as well

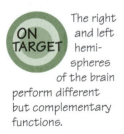

ON TARGET The right and left hemispheres of the brain perform different but complementary functions.

as playing a role in physiological regulation and serving as a relay mechanism to other parts of the brain.

Communication in the brain takes place via neuronal pathways through the conduction of electrical impulses through the neuron to its axonal endings, where the electrical stimulus results in the release of neurotransmitters into the synapse between the axon of one neuron and the dendrites of the next. The neurotransmitters either stimulate or inhibit the receiving neuron. The brain processes a multitude of stimuli simultaneously and at various levels, both consciously and unconsciously. These simultaneous processes allow for linkage of sensory, motor, cognitive, and emotional stimuli in memory. There is evidence that the brain remains plastic, or moldable, throughout life and is structurally changed at the molecular level by exposure to experiences (Howard Hughes Medical Institute 2002; Diamond 2002). Although it is not clear how it occurs, it appears that memory involves a permanent (or at least long-term) change in neural functioning through changes in the microarchitechture of the cerebral cortex (Diamond 2002; Blanchard and Thacker 1999). These findings suggest that experiences not only result in learning, but also increase the capacity to learn. This is consistent with the theoretical construct of schema formation and reorganization.

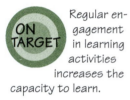

Regular engagement in learning activities increases the capacity to learn.

PEARLS Stimulating questions cause synapses in the brain to make more connections because of the mind's need to deal with the question. When reading this text, for example, if you convert this section heading into a question—What are the neurobiological considerations in learning?—you are likely to learn more than if you just read the section heading.

sensory memory
The form of memory that holds information from sensory stimulation long enough for it to be processed by working memory.

working memory
The memory structure where information processing occurs.

Changes in brain structure and function impact the ability to selectively attend to stimuli and thus interfere with learning. One example of this is attention-deficit hyperactivity disorder. Other disorders, such as dyslexia and related disorders, affect the ability to receive and process information. The ability to store and retrieve information may be affected by traumatic brain injury or Alzheimer's disease. Schizophrenia involves a variety of disorders of information processing. These phenomena allow us to appreciate the neurobiological bases of learning.

Cognition and Memory

Memory function is essential for learning. It is generally held that we use sensory; short-term, or working, memory; and long-term memory. **Sensory memory** refers to the mental maps we have for physical stimuli and movements associated with activities. For example, you don't have to think about the motions needed to bring a fork to your mouth or tie your shoes. This is referred to as kinesthetic imprinting, which can serve as a foundation to more concrete learning. We are primarily concerned here with short-term and long-term memory functions and structures. For our purposes, we use the term **working memory,** because it more accurately reflects the processing of information, rather than implying a simple storage of information. As you will soon see, the processes and structure of memory are critical considerations in instructional design.

Working Memory

Cognitive psychology theorists propose that working memory has two components. One component acts as a "scratch pad" for visual information (Sweller, van Merrienboer, and Paas 1998) and is sometimes referred to as **iconic memory.** The other component of working memory is used to temporarily hold verbal and auditory stimuli. This feature has been described by Baddeley (1992) as a **phonological loop** and is also called **echoic memory.** These two components can be thought of as partially independent information processors.

Working memory contains the contents of consciousness at any given moment. We are consciously aware only of what is in our working memory. We are not conscious of what is in our long-term memory until it is brought into our working memory for comparing and contrasting with new information. Working memory is limited. We can hold only about seven items in working memory at a time. However, because some of the load of working memory is occupied by the processes of organizing and analyzing information, we can probably consider only two or three pieces of information if we must think about, rather than just store, the information (Sweller et al.). This limitation of working memory is a vital consideration in instructional design.

Long-Term Memory

Long-term memory is considered virtually limitless. Intellectual ability comes from stored knowledge of experiences, rather than from engaging in complex logical reasoning in **short-term memory.** Problem solving, then, comes not from logical reasoning but from comparison of the current problem to previously encountered problems. Although we can solve unfamiliar problems, the cognitive process by which we do this is not as efficient. This underscores the critical role of experience in learning.

Long-term memories are stored in the form of **schemata.** Schemata categorize information for storage and can be either very simple or very complex. For example, we have a schema for "fruit" that consists of lower-level schemata of "pears," "oranges," "bananas," etc. "Fruit" is a

iconic memory
The part of sensory memory that temporarily holds visual information.

phonological loop
Echoic memory.

echoic memory
The part of sensory memory that temporarily holds auditory information.

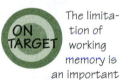 The limitation of working memory is an important consideration in instructional design and delivery.

long-term memory
The mental structure that holds schemata. We are aware of information in long-term memory only when it is pulled into working memory.

short-term memory
Working memory.

schema, schemata (pl.)
A cognitive structure that holds scripts for how things should be.

intrinsic cognitive load
The burden of information processing related to the inherent complexity of the material to be learned.

sub-schema of "food," and so on. The critical point is that no matter how complex a schema, it is considered to be a single item when it is pulled into working memory. Thus, one of the functions of schemata is to reduce the cognitive load in working memory.

Schemata also allow for automatic processing of information, further reducing the cognitive load required for conscious processing of information. These schemata can be considered "automated rules" (Sweller, Van Merrionboer, and Paas 1998). The more automated rules we have, the more working memory we have available. For example, most adults have automated the rules needed for reading. We do not have to give conscious thought to the phonetic sound represented by each letter or combination of letters as we read. Therefore, we can devote our working memory to determining the *meaning* of what is read, rather than on *how* to read. This illustrates another important concept in instructional design, which is that we need to learn simpler material and processes before we can learn more complex material.

An EMT student must learn (automate) the techniques of patient assessment before he or she will be able to effectively learn to associate the findings of the physical exam with the meaning of the findings. Otherwise, his or her working memory is overloaded with *how* to palpate, inspect, and auscultate, and there is little working memory capacity left to compare and contrast normal and abnormal findings, let alone compare the abnormal findings to the rules for specific problems. This also implies that the student must have constructed schemata for various problems to which he or she must compare the physical exam findings. As you have no doubt noticed, the novice EMT student struggles to process so much information, whereas the experienced practitioner seems to come up with a field impression almost magically. In fact, what is happening is that the experienced practitioner has formed schemata for various patient presentations and easily recognizes when a patient presentation fits a previously learned pattern. It is likely that the experienced practitioner would have to give some thought before answering if he or she were to be asked *how* he or she arrived at the conclusion.

PEARLS Organizing learning activities and content from known to unknown, simple to complex, chronologically, and in other patterns helps students build schemata. Schemata help learners recognize familiar patterns in new problems and free up working memory by creating automated rules.

Cognitive load theory also considers the effects of *intrinsic* and *extrinsic* cognitive load. **Intrinsic cognitive load** is related to the difficulty or sophistication of the material to be learned. **Extrinsic cognitive load** is

extrinsic cognitive load
Additional burden placed on information processing due to ineffective presentation of material.

the additional burden placed on working memory due to poor instructional design (Sweller, Van Merrionboer, and Paas 1998). As an educator, you cannot modify the intrinsic cognitive load of the curriculum, but you can make learning more likely through the use of effective instructional design, such as appropriate sequencing of content, in order to increase students' available working memory.

Progressivism and Constructivism in Learning

progressivism
A philosophical view that learning proceeds as we bring prior experiences to bear on future experiences.

constructivism
A theory in which learning is conceived of as constant building and refinement of knowledge structures based on experiences.

Progressivism is a larger philosophy that considers politics and other social institutions as well as education. Progressive education espouses nonauthoritarian, learner-centered, experience-based education that takes into account the diversity of people's interests and needs. This movement grew out of opposition to the traditional focus of the American public school system, which was subject-centered learning and uniformity, not diversity. Although progressivism is a philosophy of education, **constructivism** is a theory of education that fits with progressive philosophy. Constructivism proposes that we learn through continuous reconstruction of experience. We bring our prior experiences and the assumptions based on them into every new experience.

Experience alone, however, does not automatically result in learning. We must reflect on the experience and fit it in with what we already know—our existing schemata. Learning is a continual revision of our schemata. We cannot say that learning has occurred until a subsequent experience is changed by the knowledge, attitude, or skill to which the learner was previously exposed. We do not know that a student has learned something unless we see the student act in a situation in a way he or she couldn't have before. The student's knowledge of cardiology, for example, will allow him or her to recognize a dysrhythmia and act on it in a way he or she could not without knowledge of a dysrhythmia. The learning has changed the subsequent experience with the patient. Because the crux of learning is experience, you will also hear the term *experiential learning.*

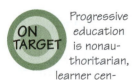 Progressive education is nonauthoritarian, learner centered, and experience based and takes into account the diversity of individuals' needs and interests.

The Effect of Prior Experience on Learning New Information

It is important to note that when we speak of constructivism, we mean that students are active constructors of their own knowledge. By the time students reach our classroom, they have constructed, through experience, a large amount of knowledge, not all of which is accurate. In many cases this knowledge is deeply rooted in the person's identity and is what he or she has relied upon for many years to make sense of the world. The previous knowledge, no matter how basic, acts as scaffolding upon which more knowledge can be built. At some point you will present information to your students that, although correct, is inconsistent (or perceived to be inconsistent) with their prior learning. As such, the new information does not fit with the students' schemata. When this occurs, students can deal with it in one of four ways (Sewell 2002). They can delete the prior knowledge, modify the prior knowledge so that the new information fits into it, modify the new information so that it fits with the existing schema, or reject the new information.

Purging old information is very difficult. Knowledge that has served us well for many years can't simply disappear or be erased. We are unlikely to discard the knowledge unless we find it is no longer sufficient to meet our needs. In fact, one of the most effective ways of getting students to see the limitations of their current beliefs is to provide a scenario in which the student's way of doing something simply will not work. Sometimes, students master regurgitating information and algorithms because they know they need to perform on an exam. But if they do not believe the accuracy of the new information, they are unlikely to remember it, let alone act on it, once they leave the classroom. Memorizing algorithms and definitions is simply a temporary storage of information, not learning. As you will recall from the beginning of the chapter, learning is a relatively permanent change in behavior (or behavior potential) that occurs due to experience. When students have simply memorized an algorithm or protocol, they will not be able to answer questions that probe the underlying principles of the algorithm. This is the essence of the much criticized "cookbook paramedic." According to Sewell, students may actually dichotomize knowledge of a particular topic such that they use one stream of knowledge in real life and the other in class and on exams.

A second option when confronted with new information that conflicts with prior learning is to modify the existing knowledge so that the new information fits into that knowledge structure. This may be more likely than completely unlearning previous knowledge, but it requires conscious effort to reconcile the inconsistent information. This is what is meant by reconstruction of experience as a result of a new experience.

A third possibility when a student is presented with new, conflicting information is to modify the new knowledge to fit the existing erroneous belief. This involves distorting the new information so that it is congruent with the existing knowledge. This is somewhat more likely because it does not involve admitting being wrong about something, which is hard for all of us to do. Yet it does involve cognitive effort, which is not always readily forthcoming. This is a very important concept in that we must be sure that what we are teaching is accurate, because once something is learned, it is very difficult to eradicate or change. Finally, when cognitive effort is not applied to reconciling inconsistent information, the new information will be rejected. This may not be readily apparent in exam performance, because "cramming" for an examination can allow the student to hold information long enough for regurgitation on an exam without actually learning the material or changing misconceptions.

Facilitating Integration of Information

As you have seen, prior learning can be a blessing or a curse in the classroom. It is not enough that you are the teacher and as such should be regarded as being "right." Although authority or expertise may serve some function, you must remember that you are competing with not only the persuasiveness of the misinformation, but also the authority and charisma of its source. Sewell suggests several ways in which we can diminish the effects of prior incorrect learning. First, you must be aware of what students' misconceptions are. With experience, you will learn to anticipate the common misconceptions that accompany students into the classroom. You can also do informal pretesting before beginning new topics to find out what students currently believe. Once you know what the misconceptions are, you can address them head-on by teaching the new information and comparing it with misconceptions (not by singling out a particular student, of course). Again, giving case studies or, even better, scenarios in which the misconception will not serve the student can be a powerful way of helping the student realize that his or her current knowledge is not adequate to solve real-life problems.

PEARLS Using scenarios and case studies in which learners' misconceptions will not work is a powerful way of allowing learners to realize that their current knowledge is inadequate to solve real-life problems.

A second important consideration is that you must avoid contributing to the misinformation. You must know your subject matter well and admit when you don't, rather than providing information of questionable validity. As mentioned earlier, once you learn something, it is extremely difficulty to erase it from memory. Additionally, know the quality and veracity of your guest instructors and instructional aids. It is important to review textbooks, workbooks, articles, "hand-me-down" presentations, and packaged instructor resources for accuracy. Obviously, some textbooks and ancillaries are better than others. But even the best products can contain a few errors or misprints, especially in their first edition, despite the best efforts of authors, editors, and reviewers. Never assign reading or homework or show video presentations that you have not reviewed.

The Importance of Reflection on Experience

It has been said that the unexamined experience is not worth having. Learning is an active process in which the learner must be cognitively engaged with experience. Immersion in information does not cause the information to seep into the brain the way water seeps into a sponge. If information is not processed in working memory, it cannot make its way into long-term memory. It is common to say that we must involve ourselves in reflection on action. This implies that we don't think about an experience until it is past. In fact, we must engage in reflection *in* action, as well. Without reflection, previous knowledge cannot be reconstructed; therefore, learning does not occur. "Courageous and creative experimentation should at the same time be responsible, which means making continuous assessments about the likely consequences and acknowledging them in action" (Kivinen and Ristela 2002, 425).

Reflection, or at least deep reflection, on experiences does not automatically occur. One of your tasks as an educator is to guide students' reflections on experiences so that they can derive meaning from activity. This is most effectively done through critical questioning and directed journaling assignments. In a later chapter you will read about specific types and examples of questioning and activities to promote student reflection.

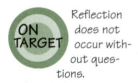

ON TARGET Reflection does not occur without questions.

Experiential Learning Models

experiential learning
Creation of knowledge through reflection on experience; deriving meaning from experiences.

It is impossible to completely capture such a complex and abstract process as learning in a simple, two-dimensional model. Nonetheless, models remain a useful way to illustrate processes, including learning. We begin with some definitions of experiential learning to provide perspective and then describe two frequently used models of experiential learning.

Experiential learning occurs through direct interaction with the phenomena of interest rather than just thinking or hearing about the experience. It involves the whole body in learning, creating a kinesthetic imprint. Experiential learning builds scaffolding for more abstract concepts. Houle (1980) describes experiential learning as education that occurs through direct participation in life events. John Dewey conceives of experiential learning as the reconstruction and reorganization of experience, which increases our ability to direct further experience. It is the construction of meaning from experience. Jarvis (1995) adds to this definition by distinguishing it as primary, or sensory, experience or secondary experience, which is reflection on the sensory experience. Experience is not complete without both aspects. Kivinen and Ristela differentiate knowing from *knowing*

ON TARGET Experiential learning is the reconstruction and reorganization of experience, which increases our ability to direct further experience. It is the construction of meaning from experience.

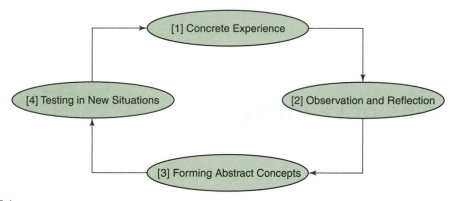

Figure 7-1
Kolb's Model of Experiential Learning
Adapted from Smith (2001). Retrieved 06/06/2003 from http://www.infed.org/biblio/b-explrn.htm.

how. "Knowing how is often tacit and cannot be reached by linguistic consciousness–the action needed to promote it cannot [only] be coded into textbooks and curricula" (2002, 424).

Kolb's model of experiential learning (Figure 7-1) is relatively straightforward and gives a useful overview of the experiential learning process. Jarvis' model (Figure 7-2) is more detailed, providing a deeper view into the learning process. Jarvis also provides an alternative pathway in which the experience provides no new information and simply reinforces existing knowledge. As you analyze these models, consider

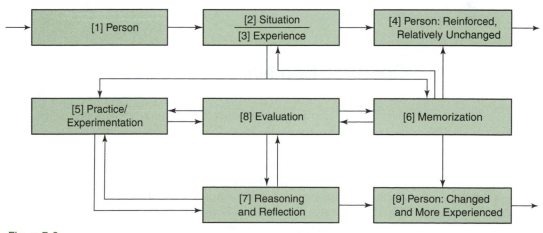

Figure 7-2
Jarvis' Model of Experiential Learning
Adapted from Smith (2001). Retrieved 06/06/2003 from http://www.infed.org/biblio/b-explrn.htm.

their application to clinical education and internships, simulations, role-play, and laboratory sessions and to projects that can be assigned as homework.

Domains of Learning

It is generally held that we learn in three different areas, or domains. The three domains of learning and the levels of complexity within them are described by Bloom's taxonomy of educational objectives (Bloom et al. 1956). Your understanding of these three domains and the levels of complexity in each is essential to your ability to write learning objectives, select the correct teaching materials and methods, and construct homework activities and quiz and exam items.

cognitive domain
The area of learning concerned with knowledge and intellectual processes.

affective domain
The area of learning concerned with values, attitudes, and emotions.

The **cognitive domain** consists of information and intellectual functions, for example, things such as reading, defining, explaining, and other mental activities. The **affective domain** consists of our attitudes and conduct and is represented by the way we behave, conduct ourselves, and treat others. The psychomotor domain consists of our bodily abilities and skills and applies to any physical action we take in carrying out our jobs. This can be somewhat confusing when we consider things such as speaking or drawing a diagram. In the EMS classroom if we ask someone to "describe" or "write" something, we are not concerned with the physical act of speaking or writing, which the students already know; we are concerned with the knowledge expressed through speaking and writing, which is in the cognitive domain. However, if we ask someone to "perform a venipuncture," we are interested in the actual manipulation of the equipment and materials by the student.

Cognitive Domain

The cognitive domain of learning is divided into the two major classes of *knowledge* and *intellectual skills and abilities*. Knowledge is the less complex of the two major classes and contains only one level within it. That level is also known as knowledge. The classification of intellectual skills and abilities contains five levels. These are, in order of increasing complexity, comprehension, application, analysis, synthesis, and evaluation. It should be noted that the various EMS NSC consolidate these six levels into only three. Level one, called *knowledge* in the NSC, corresponds to Bloom's levels 1 (knowledge) and 2 (comprehension). Level 2, called *application* in the NSC, corresponds to Bloom's level 3, application; and level 3, called *problem solving* in the

NSC, corresponds to Bloom's level 4 (analysis), level 5 (synthesis), and level 6 (evaluation).

Knowledge is simply the ability to recall previously learned material such as definitions, facts, and principles. *Comprehension* is the ability to understand the meaning of material. Level 3, *application,* refers to the ability to use information in a concrete situation. *Analysis* is the ability to break material down into its component parts, to organize it, and to identify the relationships between principles. *Synthesis* is the ability to bring together discrete parts into a whole; to construct something unique such as a treatment plan. The highest level, *evaluation,* refers to the ability to judge the value of something in a specific situation using given criteria.

Table 7-1 provides examples of actions in each of the levels of the cognitive domain.

Affective Domain

The affective domain levels are receiving, responding, valuing, organization, and characterization. *Receiving* is simply the willingness to pay attention to phenomena or stimuli. *Responding* involves active participation by student. *Valuing* refers to the importance or beliefs the student attaches to an object or behavior. *Organization* is the level at which the student resolves conflict between competing values to organize an internally consistent belief system. *Characterization* means the student can be characterized by his or her consistency and predictability in behavior.

Table 7-2 provides examples of actions in each of the levels of the affective domain.

Psychomotor Domain

The levels of complexity in the psychomotor domain include perception, set, guided response, mechanism, and complex overt response. *Perception* deals with the student's awareness of objects or qualities via the senses. *Set* refers to the mental, physical, and emotional readiness for a particular action. *Guided response* focuses on the acquisition of lower-level components of more complex tasks and includes trial and error. At the level of *mechanism,* learned responses are automatic. Abilities are combined into action of skilled nature. *Complex overt responses* are the performance of complex motor functions with a high degree of skill and efficiency. The combination of effectiveness and efficiency of action at this level is known as *proficiency*.

Table 7-3 provides examples of actions in each of the levels of the psychomotor domain.

Table 7-1   Illustrations in the Cognitive Domain

Level	Examples of Verbs Used in Cognitive Objectives	Illustrative Objective	Examples of Evaluation Appropriate to the Level of Objective
Knowledge	Define, identify, list, describe, label, match, state, select, recognize	The student should be able to list the signs and symptoms of hypoglycemia.	List four signs of hypoglycemia.
Comprehension	Distinguish, differentiate, compare and contrast, explain, generalize, give examples, summarize, interpret	The student should be able to distinguish the signs of hypoglycemia from those of hyperglycemia.	Which of the following is a sign of hypoglycemia? a. Kusmaul's respirations b. Dehydration c. Fruity breath odor d. Diaphoresis
Application	Demonstrate, modify, predict, solve, use	Given a history of the present illness, the student should be able to predict the nature of patient's condition.	Your patient took insulin this morning but has not eaten. Is the patient more likely to be hypoglycemic or hyperglycemic?
Analysis	Break down, diagram, distinguish, separate, categorize, outline, abstract	Given a scenario, the student should be able to categorize the patient's condition as life-threatening or non-life-threatening.	Your patient is unresponsive to all stimuli and has snoring respirations at 8 per minute. Would you consider your patient to be in life-threatening or non-life-threatening condition?
Synthesis	Combine, create, devise, plan, generate, develop, construct	Given a scenario, the student should be able to develop a clinical impression of the patient's problem.	Your patient has been thirsty, hungry, urinating frequently, and increasingly lethargic for 3 days. Given that the patient has diabetes, what is your impression of the problem?
Evaluation	Appraise, compare, conclude, judge, evaluate, justify, defend, critique, support, provide a rationale	Given a scenario including initial patient condition, initial interventions, and postintervention condition, the student should be able to judge the effectiveness of the treatment plan.	Your patient had an initial blood glucose level of 20 mg%. Following the administration of 25 g of dextrose, the patient is more alert and has a blood glucose level of 122 mg%. What intervention(s) should you consider next?

Table 7-2 Illustrations in the Affective Domain

Level	Examples of Verbs Used in Affective Objectives	Illustrative Objective	Examples of Evaluation Appropriate to the Level of Objective
Receiving	Acknowledge, recognize	The student should be able to recognize instances in which a patient is uncomfortable talking in front of his or her family.	Your patient is 14-year-old boy who was injured while riding personal watercraft. His parents are very anxious, but the patient is reluctant to give you a history of the event. What factors might account for this reluctance?
Responding	Reply, answer, comply, conform, demonstrate, assist	The student should be able to respond with empathy when dealing with the dying patient.	Your patient has end-stage terminal cancer and seems to be depressed. Which of the following statements would be appropriate? a. You seem sad; is there anything you would like to talk about? b. It's time for you to accept what is going to happen to you. c. I'm an EMT; it's not my job to talk to you about your feelings. d. I feel so terrible for you; I don't know how you can handle this.
Valuing	Explain, defend, justify, propose	The student should be able to explain the importance of professional conduct by the EMT.	Write a short paragraph explaining the importance of professional conduct by the EMT.
Organization	Integrate, organize, decide	Given a situation in which the patient's wishes conflict with those of the family, the student should be able decide upon an ethical course of action.	Your patient is a 68-year-old man dying of cancer. His family called the ambulance, but the patient, who is alert and oriented, states his wish is to die at home. The family is nearly hysterical, insisting that you do everything you can and transport the patient to the hospital. Explain how you will handle this situation.
Characterization	Act, display, influence	The student will display professional demeanor at all times.	This can best be assessed by clinical preceptors and would be appropriate for inclusion in student clinical evaluation.

Table 7-3   Illustrations in the Psychomotor Domain

Level	Examples of Verbs Used in Psychomotor Objectives	Illustrative Objective	Examples of Evaluation Appropriate to the Level of Objective
Perception	Recognizes, identifies, palpates, auscultates, inspects	The student should be able to recognize the Korotkoff sounds when auscultating a blood pressure.	This could best be evaluated by the use of a teaching stethoscope, asking the student to indicate when he or she hears the changes in the character of the sounds.
Set	Prepares, lays out, assembles, selects, positions	The student should be able to correctly position the patient for a log roll.	This is best evaluated by direct observation using a set of criteria for judging the student's performance.
Guided response	Imitates, manipulates, applies, measures, discovers	Given a scenario in which a patient is unresponsive in a vehicle, the student should be able to discover the best way to remove the patient from the vehicle.	This is best evaluated by observing scenario performance.
Mechanism	Applies, inserts, administers, calibrates	The student should be able to apply a properly fitting cervical collar.	This is best evaluated by observing and checking against criteria for performance.
Complex overt response	Drives, performs, intubates	The student should be able to intubate the trachea under direct laryngoscopy in less than 30 seconds.	This is best evaluated by observation of student performance, making sure all critical steps are completed.

Summary

Learning is a complex process that is not yet completely understood. In this chapter you have read about the neurobiological bases of learning and the concept of brain plasticity. You have also been introduced to the concepts of working memory and long-term memory. Working memory is limited and is where we consciously process information, whereas long-term memory is virtually limitless and stores information from experiences in schematic form. All learning takes place through experience, though not all experiences are educative. We construct our identity through our experiences, making the knowledge gained from experiences very powerful. These prior experiences can either act as scaffolding for further experiences or can cause rejection of inconsistent information. Reflection on experiences allows a continuous reconstruction of experience—we both bring something into and take something with us from every experience. That experience is the basis for the ability to direct subsequent experience illustrates the progressive, constructive nature of learning. There are three types of learning, referred to as domains. The cognitive domain deals with knowledge and rational thought. The affective domain deals with our attitudes, values, and beliefs; and the psychomotor domain refers to bodily-kinesthetic learning. Understanding these domains is critical to creating learning objectives, guiding us in the selection of teaching-learning methods and determining the best ways to write exam items.

REVIEW QUESTIONS

1. What is the essence of constructivism as a theory of education?

2. In which domain of learning would you categorize this objective: The learner should be able to create a written examination?

3. What is the role of experience in learning?

4. Describe the three domains of learning.

5. What activities can you, as an instructor, use to stimulate learners to reflect on experience?

Overview of the Educational Planning and Curriculum- Development Processes

Learning Objectives

Upon completion of this chapter you should be able to

- Define curriculum.

- Discuss the components of a curriculum.

- Define competency-based education.

- Utilize a planning model for curriculum development.

- Use the current EMS National Standard Curricula to plan programs.

- Discuss how the use of the educational standards that will replace current NSC will impact the program-planning and curriculum-development processes.

- Employ a systematic approach to program planning.

CASE
Study_____

Lieutenant Ron Stiles, the Dixon Township Fire Department EMS training coordinator, has been asked by his captain to develop a training session for firefighter/paramedic Greg Davies. Earlier in the week paramedic Davies had made two unsuccessful attempts to intubate a trauma patient with a closed head injury. Davies managed the patient's airway by BLS means and transported her to the trauma center. Upon arrival at the trauma center, the patient received medications for rapid sequence induction of anesthesia and was successfully intubated.

Questions

1. Is this a situation that requires educational intervention?
2. How would you go about determining if educational intervention is warranted?
3. Aside from an educational intervention, what actions might be appropriate?

Introduction

The planning function of educational programs is a critical, but often overlooked, activity in the educational endeavor. Lack of systematic planning results in educational offerings that do not meet the needs of learners and stakeholders, thus wasting time and money. The effects can be far-reaching, impacting the reputation of the institution. Currently, we rely on very prescriptive EMS NSCs that specify objectives, minimum declarative material, and the suggested time frames for the lessons. As the current NSC are replaced with less-detailed educational standards, the need for skilled program planners will be great. This chapter discusses program and curriculum planning in the context of competency-based education and differentiates between program planning for preservice or primary EMS education and planning for continuing professional development activities.

KEY TERMS

accreditation, p. 122

advisory committee, p. 122

community of interest, p. 122

competency-based education (CBE), p. 121

curriculum, curricula (pl.), p. 119

descriptive curriculum, p. 123

What Is a Curriculum?

**curriculum,
curricula (pl.)**
The interrelationship between the purpose of a program of education, the functions the program will serve, and the structure and processes used to achieve the program's purpose.

The essence of a **curriculum** lies in the interrelationships between the purpose of a program of education, the functions the program serves, and the structure and processes used to achieve the program's purpose. A curriculum is more than a series of courses or the prescribed content of an educational program. The outcome of a curriculum is greater than the sum of the individual classes or modules in it. Ralph Tyler (1949) proposes that curriculum development is accomplished by studying four questions, using a systematic process to formulate answers to them. The four questions to be considered in curriculum development are

1. What educational purposes (goals and objectives) are we seeking to attain?

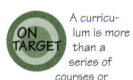

A curriculum is more than a series of courses or prescribed content of a program. A curriculum addresses the relationships between the purposes of the program, the functions it will serve, and the structures and processes used to reach its goals.

2. How can learning experiences be selected which are likely to be useful in attaining these purposes?

3. How can these experiences be organized for effective learning?

4. How can the effectiveness of these experiences be evaluated?

According to Prideaux, " . . . the curriculum should achieve a 'symbiosis' with the health services and communities in which the students will serve. The values that underlie the curriculum should enhance health service provision. The curriculum must be responsive to changing values and expectations in education if it is to remain useful" (2003, 268).

Review of Educational Concepts

learning
A constant reconstruction of knowledge through reflection on experience.

It is helpful here to review some of the basic concepts covered previously so that we can consider the relationship between *education, teaching, teacher,* and *learning* in the processes of program and curriculum development. **Learning**, at its most basic level, is a relatively permanent change in behavior as a result of experience. **Teaching** refers to the instruction or contribution to the development of others by skillfully arranging learning experiences. A **teacher** is a person employed to guide and direct the experiences of students. **Education** is the sum of all

processes through which a person develops abilities, aptitudes, and other forms of behavior of a positive value to the society in which he or she lives. In this sense, education refers to both formal and informal education. Formal education can be viewed as a social process by which people are subjected to the influence of a selected environment so that they may become socially competent and reach optimum personal development (Dewey 1938). In planning a curriculum or instructional program, it is important to have a clear idea of (1) who the learners are, (2) what the needs of society are, and (3) what the best ways of bringing about learning and development are in order to deliver an educational product.

Competency-based Education

teaching
Arranging the conditions under which learning occurs.

EMS education is competency based in that the tasks of the occupation are prespecified. Education is directed at student achievement of these competencies. According to Seibert (1979), **competency-based education (CBE)** focuses on preparing students to perform the prespecified competencies of a profession under real-life conditions at a level of proficiency required of workers on the job. The four components of CBE are behavior statements (objectives), subject matter content, opportunities for learning, and evaluation.

A competency is a statement of expected behavior that includes the conditions of performance and standards of acceptable performance. These are broad statements also known as terminal performance objectives (TPO). A curriculum contains objectives, or competencies, in all three domains of learning. Because competencies must reflect the real-life content and conditions of jobs, they are derived from **job analyses.** You can find the Functional Job Analysis for paramedics as an appendix to the paramedic NSC (NHTSA 1998). The NREMT has also published a Practice Analysis for NREMT-Bs, NREMT-Is, and NREMT-Ps (NREMT 2005).

Components of a Curriculum

teacher
A person employed to guide the experiences of learners to result in learning.

A curriculum document contains specific information that is used for program-approval processes and accreditation purposes and to ensure continuity and consistency in the educational program. The development of the curriculum should be preceded by a needs analysis and feasibility study to establish the need for the program and whether or not the resources needed to conduct the program can be obtained.

The curriculum document begins with a statement of *program purpose and goals*. This is a brief discussion that provides background and context to support the need for the program as well as a very specific statement of the purpose and a listing of the program-level goals. This statement should make it clear that there is need for this particular program by discussing what is unique about it. For example, will the program fill a geographical void, meet demand that cannot be met by existing programs, or offer a unique program of studies not otherwise available in the area?

The curriculum contains a *philosophy statement* that describes the philosophical influences on curriculum development. This is an essential part of the document that allows the reader to interpret the curriculum within the intended framework. This statement might reflect the philosophical beliefs related to progressive education, for example. In addition, it is essential that the philosophy of a curriculum developed within an institution reflect the mission of the institution. When proposing a new curriculum in a college or university setting, it is necessary to demonstrate how the curriculum contributes to the mission of the institution.

A description of the student *population to be served* provides additional framework for interpretation of the curriculum. If the intended audience for a program is new high school graduates, the curriculum might be different than if the intended audience is a group of English as a second language (ESL) adults. This information is also important in effective marketing of the program.

The *curriculum overview* briefly describes the program of study, providing a sample student program plan, and any curriculum prerequisites. This is simply a listing of course titles, numbers, and credit hours, if applicable, in the sequence that the courses would normally be taken. Following this, a more-detailed list of *course titles and descriptions* is provided. Educational institutions generally have conventions for course numbering, course titles, and the assignment of credit hours. Commonly, course numbering in four-year colleges and universities uses three digits. The course numbers that begin with zero, such as EMS 080, denote a prerequisite or remedial class, such as CPR. The 100-level courses correspond to freshman-level courses, the 200-level courses correspond to sophomore-level courses, and so on. There is also usually a convention for assigning section numbers to courses. The assignment of course credits generally goes by a rule similar to the following: lecture classes receive a one-to-one ratio of clock hours to credit hours, so that a class that meets for 3 hours a week for one semester receives three credit hours. For a laboratory course the ratio is 1 credit hour per 2 clock hours, and for a clinical course the ratio is generally 1 credit hour per 3 clock hours. You will need to follow the conventions of your institution and guidelines established by the commission on higher education in your state, where applicable.

The next section of the curriculum document is a list of the *terminal performance objectives for each course* in the program. The more-detailed enabling objectives will be a part of the lesson plans for individual course sessions, which are not typically found in the curriculum document. This list describes the breadth and depth of the content of each course and allows for the discovery of gaps and areas of overlap between courses. The formation of a matrix cross-referencing the program competencies with the course terminal performance objectives helps identify any overlap or gaps.

Faculty credentials are included, as well. These state the minimum instructor requirements for each course in the program. Considerations include professional experience, educational credentials, and educational background area(s). A list of *required clinical affiliations* is included, as well. This list should be created with consideration of the skill competencies (IVs, endotracheal intubations, patient assessments, etc.) stated in the NSC and whether each agency or institution can provide enough patient contact in the required areas in a reasonable amount of time for the number of students projected to be enrolled in the program.

An **advisory committee** is a necessary part of your program and should consist of **stakeholders** and advisors to your program. These individuals ideally have had an opportunity to provide input to the curriculum committee during the curriculum-development process and should meet two to three times per year. An advisory committee may consist of 5 to 10 or so individuals whose guidance and input is critical to your program. Your institution may have specific guidelines for the composition of advisory committees. The advisory committee or council should be representative of the demographic composition of the area in age and ethnicity and should have sufficient representation of males and females. There should be representatives from **communities of interest,** such as the public health department, potential employers, emergency physician groups, the public, area EMS council, and local hospital commission. There should also be representation from professionals who can provide guidance in important areas, such as course content, evaluation, and legal matters.

Newly created programs do not have the data necessary for a self-study in preparation for **accreditation** by the CoAEMSP but may be able to attain provisional accreditation. If the curriculum is for a newly created program, the accreditation section should include concrete plans for attaining accreditation. This section should also list any accrediting bodies for the institution.

advisory committee
An organized body of individuals that provides consultation and guidance to a program.

stakeholder
A party with an interest in the operation and outcomes of an entity.

community of interest
A group with a stake in the program outcomes.

accreditation
The process of certifying that an institution meets prescribed standards.

The operating *budget* for your program is important for the curriculum-approval process as well. You will need to use an approved budget format to project funding, revenues, and expenses for your program. One of the purposes of the budget is to predict when the program will be self-sustaining and, in many institutions, profitable. Finally, you will include a list of any *references* you used during the curriculum-development process. Remember, your institution may have specific requirements for the curriculum document.

Curriculum Planning Models

prescriptive curriculum
A detailed, directive program of instruction.

descriptive curriculum
A curriculum stated as the context, needs, and values related to the program, rather than using a directive approach.

The two major "pure" classifications of curriculum-planning models are **prescriptive** and **descriptive curricula.** The EMS national standard curricula with which we work are prescriptive. They are concerned with outcomes, or competencies, and are objective based. Outcomes-based models guide curriculum development from the desired outcomes backward. The essential thought behind this is that we have to know where we are going before we can decide how to get there. With this in mind, it is important to remember that we do curricular planning with evaluation in mind. We must know how we will know that the outcomes have been achieved.

Descriptive models are more concerned with describing the context, or situation, of a curriculum. Factors to be considered include the expectations of society and employers, the nature of the occupation, available support and resources, students, the institution, and problems existing with the way things are currently being done (e.g., low registry exam pass rates, attrition, etc.). In reality, both the prescriptive and descriptive elements of curriculum planning should be used in EMS. The NSC or educational standards are prescriptive, but your program exists in a unique community and institution that must be considered.

Figure 8-1 provides an example of a model based on an interpretation of Tyler's principles of curriculum development. Figure 8-2 provides an example of a systems model of curriculum development.

Program and Course Planning

Program and course planning take place on a much smaller scale and often have curricula or guidelines in place to guide their development. As with a curriculum, a program, whether a 1-day seminar or a

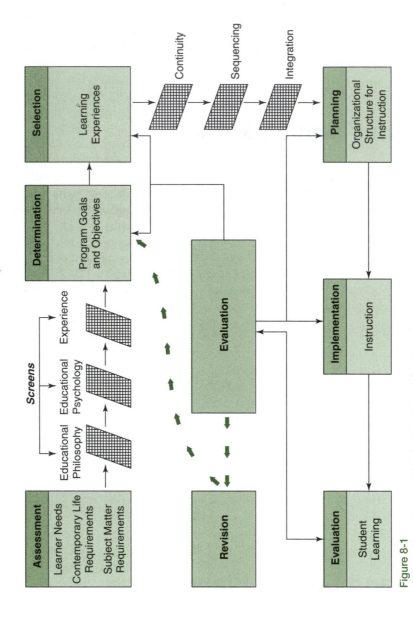

Figure 8-1

Model Interpretation of Tyler's Principles of Curriculum

Dr. Karen E. Gable, Dept. Chr., Health Sciences, School of Health & Rehabilitation Sciences, Indiana University.

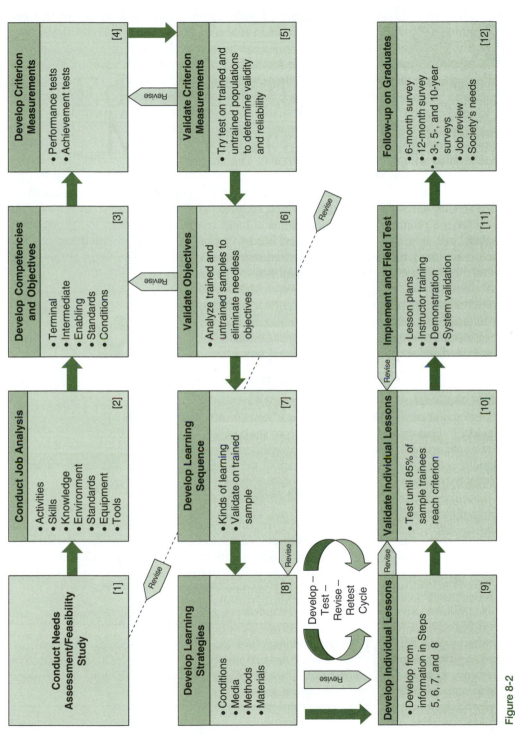

Conduct Needs Assessment/Feasibility Study [1]

Conduct Job Analysis [2]
- Activities
- Skills
- Knowledge
- Environment
- Standards
- Equipment
- Tools

Develop Competencies and Objectives [3]
- Terminal
- Intermediate
- Enabling
- Standards
- Conditions

Develop Criterion Measurements [4]
- Performance tests
- Achievement tests

Validate Criterion Measurements [5]
- Try test on trained and untrained populations to determine validity and reliability

Validate Objectives [6]
- Analyze trained and untrained samples to eliminate needless objectives

Develop Learning Sequence [7]
- Kinds of learning
- Validate on trained sample

Develop Learning Strategies [8]
- Conditions
- Media
- Methods
- Materials

Develop Individual Lessons [9]
- Develop from information in Steps 5, 6, 7, and 8

Validate Individual Lessons [10]
- Test until 85% of sample trainees reach criterion

Implement and Field Test [11]
- Lesson plans
- Instructor training
- Demonstration
- System validation

Follow-up on Graduates [12]
- 6-month survey
- 12-month survey
- 3-, 5-, and 10-year surveys
- Job review
- Society's needs

Revise

Develop – Test – Revise – Retest Cycle

Figure 8-2
Systems Model of Curriculum Planning
Adapted from unknown source.

125

12-week class, is planned with evaluation in mind. The steps in a systematic program-planning process include a needs analysis, determination of outcomes and objectives, development of course content, selection of teaching methods, and evaluation. Evaluation should be both *formative* and *summative* and should focus on both students and the program. Formative evaluation is the assessment of participants and the effectiveness of the program while the program is being conducted. Summative evaluation refers to the "final" outcomes of the students and impact of the program. Revision necessarily follows evaluation in order to keep the program on track toward the intended outcomes.

Caffarella's interactive model of program planning consists of 11 steps suited for planning continuing-education programs. Although in many cases, the essential content of continuing-education programs in EMS may be predetermined by state regulations, the delivery of these programs still requires planning and creativity. The steps of the model are as follows (1994, 18):

- Establish a basis for the planning process.
- Identify program ideas.
- Sort and prioritize program ideas.
- Develop program objectives.
- Prepare for the transfer of learning.
- Formulate evaluation plans.
- Determine formats, schedules, and staff needs.
- Prepare budgets and marketing plans.
- Design instructional plans.
- Coordinate facilities.
- Communicate the value of the program.

It should be noted that in most cases in EMS, in order for participants to obtain continuing-education credits, the program would need to be approved by the appropriate state agency and/or CECBEMS. You will need to follow the guidelines of these organizations for the submission of applications and course outlines.

Needs Analysis

needs analysis
A systematic collec-
tion of information
to determine targets
for education.

Needs analysis is an essential step in making sure your program meets a true educational need. Even when continuing-education requirements are relatively structured, there is room for flexibility to meet the specific needs of your audience. The first step in planning an educational offering is to make sure that the problem toward which it is targeted is a problem that can be solved by education. Often, managers suggest a training program to address a problem that is not, in fact, the result of a knowledge or skill deficit. In times of organizational turmoil, education is also often seen as "the answer" when there are most likely deeper underlying problems that need to be addressed.

Donaldson and Scannell (1986, 23) suggest the following methods of performing a needs analysis:

- Informal interview (conversations with employees, supervisors, managers).
- Observation of people on the job.
- Surveys.
- Performance tests.
- Formal interviews.
- Reports from superiors (especially applicable for targeted individual remedial education).
- Examination of records (CQI should be linked to continuing education).
- Advisory committees (perhaps a group of employees and supervisors).
- Formal research.

When conducting a needs analysis, it is useful to use more than one method to verify needs. Often, what people think they need to know is not really where the knowledge deficit lies. For example, a survey of employees might reveal that they believe they need 12-lead EKG training, when the results of CQI indicate there is a problem with basic lead-II rhythm interpretation. A variety of problems, such as unclear expectations or policies, can lead supervisory staff to believe there is a training problem, when all that is needed is some clarification. Throwing training at these types of problems is expensive and ineffective. The Mager analysis (Mager and Pipe 1997) is an excellent and quickly applied flowchart-type tool that can help differentiate between different types of performance problems. It asks a series of questions designed to define the problem, explore its causes, and suggest ways to address the problem. See Figure 8-3 for an overview of the Mager analysis.

Figure 8-3
Overview of the Mager
Analysis
Adapted from Mager and
Pipe (1997).

Step 1: What is the problem? Whose performance is in question? What exactly is the discrepancy between the way things are and the way things are supposed to be?

Step 2: Is the problem worth addressing? For example, is it a personal preference or is the presence of the problem consequential to the desired outcomes?

Step 3: Is this problem caused by factors other than lack of knowledge or skill? Are the following in place?
• Clear expectations for performance.
• Adequate resources available.
• Awareness of the quality of his or her performance.

Step 4: What are the consequences of the individual's or individuals' performance?
• Is the desired performance punishing? For example, if the individual is good at a particular task, is he or she being overwhelmed by increased expectations of performing that task?
• Is poor performance rewarding?
• Are there any consequences for performance at all? For example, are there ways in which employees are recognized for their contributions?

Step 5: If the problem has not been discovered at one of the earlier steps, there may be a true skill or knowledge deficiency.
• Has the person ever been able to perform the task?
• How frequently is the task performed?

Step 6: Is the task or process unnecessarily complicated? Can it be made simpler? For example, if an ambulance crew has repeatedly had an insufficient number of long backboards upon inspection of their vehicle, is it because they don't know better or don't care? Or could it be that the procedure for obtaining equipment (of any kind) is arduous or faulty?

Step 7: Are there any other barriers related to good job performance?

Step 8: Does the person have the potential to change? If yes, then training is warranted.

Summary

The key to efficient and effective educational programs is engaging in a systematic process of planning. Curriculum planning is a macro-process that guides the construction, implementation, and evaluation of an entire program of study. Program planning takes place on a smaller scale but is no less important. Effective planning makes the difference between successful and unsuccessful educational programs.

REVIEW QUESTIONS

1. Differentiate between prescriptive and descriptive curricula.

2. List at least four sources of information for an educational needs analysis.

3. When developing a continuing education program, at what point are the objectives determined?

4. List at least four of the components of a curriculum document.

5. From what source of information should curriculum competencies be derived?

Determining and Communicating Educational Needs

Learning Objectives

Upon completion of this chapter you should be able to

- Explain the importance of conducting a needs analysis/assessment for an educational program.

- Explain the importance of conducting job/occupational/ practice analysis as the basis for determining professional competencies.

- Explain the importance of using a task analysis when teaching psychomotor skills.

- Conduct a needs analysis/assessment for an educational program.

- Conduct a task analysis for a given EMS skill.

- Explain the purpose of preparing a training proposal.

- Prepare a training proposal.

CASE Study _____

Jillian Zachary has been hired as a consultant to the Waterloo Critical Care Transport Service to develop a plan for employee training and development for the next fiscal year. She will be meeting with the company's top administrators in 45 days to discuss her findings and recommendations.

Questions

1. What is the starting point for Jillian's project?
2. What type of information will she need in order to develop conclusions and make recommendations?
3. How can she collect information?
4. How should she communicate her findings and recommendations to the company decision makers?

Introduction

In the last chapter you learned about curriculum and program planning as macrolevel processes to ensure that educational programming is relevant and organized. In this chapter, we go into more detail concerning some of the processes related to curriculum and program planning. This chapter presents the details of job analysis, needs analysis, and task analysis, which will help you determine and communicate educational needs.

KEY TERMS

job analysis, p. 132

needs analysis, p. 146

occupational analysis, p. 133

performance gap, p. 146

practice analysis, p. 133

training proposal, p. 146

Job Analysis

job analysis
Systematic collection of data to define the tasks of a job, the knowledge and skills required for the job, and the context in which the tasks are performed.

Job analysis is also referred to as **occupational analysis** and **practice analysis,** although Raymond (2001) makes a good argument that practice analysis is narrower in scope than job or occupational analysis. Harvey defines job analysis as ". . . the collection of data describing (a) observable (or otherwise verifiable) job behaviors performed by workers, including both what is accomplished as well as what technologies are employed to accomplish the end results and (b) verifiable characteristics of the job environment with which workers interact, including physical, mechanical, social, and informational elements" (1991, 74). One of the purposes of job analysis is to collect evidence against which to measure the validity of educational competencies and standardized certification exams (Raymond). Job analysis is also the basis for creating job descriptions and job classifications. The 1998 Paramedic NSC (NHTSA 1998) is based on a functional job analysis conducted by the United States Department of Labor. The National Registry examination test plans are based on practice analyses of each level of certification. It is important to be familiar with these practice analyses because they are the basis of standardized testing. However, because of regional, state, and local differences in what EMS providers do, it may be a good idea to conduct a job analysis to determine if the NSC meets the needs of area EMS providers.

> **PEARLS** The current NSC and National Registry of EMTs exams are based on separate analyses of the tasks and knowledge of EMS providers.

Methods of job analysis include task inventories, generally in questionnaire format, professional performance situation models, critical incident studies, and functional job analysis. Job analyses collect information about the knowledge, skills, and abilities (KSAs) needed by job incumbents, and often classify these KSAs in terms of the frequency, risk, criticality, and other elements of the task.

Task Analysis

Although the tasks of an occupation are defined by the job analysis, a task analysis is necessary to break a task down into its discrete elements. Essentially, it is a process of decomposition of the task. Decomposition is an important step in determining the enabling objectives of a task and in discovering the teaching steps involved in teaching the task. This activity is consistent with principles of effective learning in that we must understand each step of the task and approach the task elements from simple to complex. Task analyses may be performed for either cognitive or psychomotor tasks, and there will nearly always be some requisite cognitive knowledge involved in psychomotor tasks (Militello and Hutton 1998). Task analysis is a valuable tool in teaching because as experts in the task, educators often omit details that seem implicit. These steps are assumed because we have automated the tasks over many repetitions, yet they must be made explicit to the novice. This concept often becomes clear when you attempt to explain the steps in doing something as seemingly simple such as tying your shoes or making a peanut butter and jelly sandwich. You will find that if your "student" follows your

ON TARGET Task analysis is a process of decomposing a task into its most basic steps.

instructions to the letter as if he or she did not know how to perform the task that you will probably not get the results you anticipated, even though you thought you were very clear in your explanation.

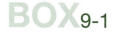 **PEARLS** Task analysis is a valuable activity for EMS educators, because we often are so familiar with skills that we perform them unconsciously and often leave out critical information needed by novices.

Rarely in EMS do we find resources that break tasks down to a level suitable for use in teaching. Skill evaluation sheets generally list only the critical aspects of a task, not the substeps within the task. One simple way of decomposing a task is to construct a task diagram or flow sheet. Another way is to use a set of index cards or Post-it Notes™, writing on each the main step and the prerequisite condition for the task. The cards or notes can then be easily arranged and rearranged as additional steps are considered. The steps in conducting a task analysis are listed in Box 9-1. Box 9-2 gives a detailed task analysis for endotracheal intubation.

BOX 9-1

Steps in Performing a Task Analysis

- Prepare a card for each element of the task.
  - List the preceding condition (stimulus).
  - Write the verb describing the action to be taken (this will become an enabling objective).
  - List the time, observation, and preparation for each step.
  - Write the justification or rationale for each step.
- Arrange the cards in sequential order, which may be linear or branching, depending on the nature of the task.
  - For branching steps, there must be a card advising that there is a discrimination, or decision to be made.
- Use the arrangement of cards to write the task instructions. The card layout indicates the major headings, subheadings, and discrimination headings.
- Evaluate the analysis. Have someone unfamiliar with the task try it out following the steps exactly as written. When the trainee makes a mistake, clarify the instructions or add steps as necessary.

BOX 9-2

Sample Task Analysis

SKILL: Endotracheal intubation under direct laryngoscopy (adult patient).

CRITERIA:
- *Without interruption of patient ventilation for greater than 30 seconds.*
- Without preventable trauma to the patient.
- With equipment and procedures suited to the individual patient.

STIMULUS AND CONTEXT: Assessment of airway and breathing reveals inadequate ventilation and/or inability of patient to maintain a patent airway in the absence of immediately correctable causes (hypoglycemia, narcotic overdose) and in the absence of the need to immediately defibrillate the patient or to move to a safer location. This task analysis assumes an unresponsive patient without a gag reflex. For patients who are responsive or who have a gag reflex yet who still require intubation, the use of topical anesthetics, medication-assisted intubation, or rapid sequence induction (RSI) may be desirable, per local protocol. It is also assumed that there is not a likelihood of cervical spine injury.

RATIONALE: Endotracheal intubation is the definitive method of isolating the airway for ventilation, prevention of gastric distention, and protection from aspiration of gastric contents, blood, or other materials. Endotracheal intubation allows for sustained airway management via mechanical ventilation. Endotracheal intubation also establishes a means for the administration of selected medications in the absence of intravenous access.

PREREQUISITE KSAs:

1. Performs manual airway maneuvers (e.g., head-tilt/chin-lift, jaw thrust).
2. Inserts basic airway adjuncts (oropharyngeal and nasopharyngeal airways).
3. Performs ventilation via bag-valve-mask device.
4. Administers supplemental oxygen.

5. Identifies structures of the airway.
6. Explains the physiology of ventilation and respiration.
7. Recognizes indications and contraindications for endotracheal intubation.
8. Anticipates complications of endotracheal intubation.
9. Values the role of endotracheal intubation in providing superior airway management, ventilation, and oxygenation.

SKILL OVERVIEW:

1. Employ appropriate level of BSI.
2. Provide initial ventilation and oxygenation.
3. Assemble needed equipment.
4. Prepare and check equipment.
5. Position yourself and your equipment.
6. Interrupt ventilation.
7. Position the patient.
8. Employ Sellick maneuver.
9. Visualize glottis.
10. Place endotracheal tube.
11. Verify correct placement of endotracheal tube.
12. Ventilate patient.
13. Secure tube.
14. Continue evaluation of ventilatory adequacy and oxygenation.

SKILL TERMINUS:

The skill of intubation is completed when correct tube placement is confirmed and the endotracheal tube is secured. Ongoing assessment of ventilation and oxygenation continues until the patient is transferred to a facility for ongoing care.

Task Analysis

Primary Step	Subcomponents	Notes
1. Employ appropriate level of BSI.	**a.** Mask **b.** Eye protection **c.** Gloves **d.** Gown if indicated	*Rationale:* Endotracheal intubation may precipitate vomiting or coughing of potentially infectious material.
2. Provide initial ventilation and oxygenation.	**a.** Manual positioning **b.** Basic airway adjunct **c.** Suctioning, if needed **d.** Bag-valve-mask ventilation **e.** Addition of supplemental oxygen	*Rationale:* Preexisting hypoxia must be corrected to mitigate tissue hypoxia and the possibility of pharyngeal stimulation induced cardiac arrhythmias. *Notes:* Ventilation and oxygenation must not be delayed to prepare for intubation. Ideally, initial ventilation and oxygenation will be provided by one or more assistants.
3. Assemble needed equipment.	**a.** Laryngoscope handle and blade **b.** Endotracheal tube **c.** Syringe **d.** Stylet (optional) **e.** Securing device **f.** Suction supplies **g.** Stethoscope **h.** Adjunctive placement verification devices **i.** Availability of bag-valve device and supplemental oxygen, as in Step 2	*Rationale:* All equipment must be at hand in order to minimize delays in tube placement once the procedure is begun.

Task Analysis (continued)

Primary Step	Subcomponents	Notes
4. Prepare and check equipment.	**a.** Insert laryngoscope blade into handle: • Hold handle in nondominant hand with bar upward and turned toward the dominant hand. • Hold blade in dominant hand with receiving groove end upward and turned toward nondominant hand. • Holding the handle and blade parallel to each other, place receiving groove of the blade over the bar and pull the blade downward until it clicks into place. • Elevate the blade to a 90° angle with respect to the handle until it locks into place. **b.** Check laryngoscope bulb. • Check to see if the bulb is illuminated with a steady, white light. • Turn bulb unit clockwise to ensure it is secured.	*Rationale:* Equipment must be determined to be safe and in working order to eliminate time delays once the procedure is begun. *Notes:* This is the mechanism by which electrical contact is made in order to light the bulb. The bulb must be bright and steady in order to illuminate the anatomical structures visualized during laryngoscopy. A loose bulb may not make sufficient contact to light and may present an aspiration hazard to the patient; at the least, it will cause a time delay for replacement if it should become lost. Conserve the batteries and bulb of the laryngoscope until ready for use.

c. Lower laryngoscope blade until ready to proceed with Step 9.

d. Check patency of the endotracheal tube cuff.

Once a patient is intubated, extubation and reintubation because of a faulty cuff will result in less-than-optimal airway management. A faulty cuff does not protect the lower airway.

- Open endotracheal tube packaging, protecting the distal tip from contamination.
- Fill the syringe with 10 mL of air.
- Attach the syringe to the inflation port of the endotracheal tube.
- Inflate the cuff and observe for leaks.
- Pull on the plunger of the syringe to evacuate the cuff and leave the syringe (filled with air) attached to the inflation port.

This keeps the syringe available and ready for inflating the cuff once the tube is placed.

e. If the use of a stylet is desired, place it through the proximal end of the endotracheal tube, ensuring that the tip of the stylet is recessed 0.5 to 1 cm into the distal end of the tube.

Often, endotracheal tubes are too flexible to successfully navigate the anatomy of the airway. The use of a stylet adds rigidity to the tube and allows the distal tip to be angled anteriorly in the airway to facilitate passage through the glottis.

f. Use the stylet to slightly bend the distal end of the endotracheal tube into a "hockey stick" curve.

Task Analysis (continued)

Primary Step	Subcomponents	Notes
5. Position yourself at the patient's head and place all needed equipment within reach.		*Note:* There are varying positions that may be assumed in order to efficiently intubate. Some factors to consider are • Location of and access to the patient. • Personal preference.
6. Interrupt bag-valve mask ventilation and chest compressions.		*Note:* Ventilation should not be interrupted for more than 30 s. Ideally, have an assistant time this interval. Alternatively, hold your breath at this point. When you need to take a breath, so does your patient.
7. Quickly but gently position the patient's neck in moderate hyperextension.	a. Place the dominant hand on the patient's forehead and push downward. b. Simultaneously, place the nondominant hand under the patient's mandible and elevate the chin.	*Rationale:* This provides alignment of the airway anatomy into the line of vision. *Note:* A towel roll may be used beneath the patient's shoulders to assist in maintaining this position; alternatively, an assistant may stabilize the head in this position.
8. Ask an assistant to provide cricoid pressure (Sellick maneuver).	See task analysis for this skill.	*Rationale:* Reduces chances of aspiration of gastric contents during intubation and may assist in bringing the glottis into view.

9. Visualize the glottis.

c. Hold the handle of the laryngoscope in the left hand and elevate the blade to a 90° angle.

d. Perform a tongue-jaw lift with the right hand.

e. Insert the tip of the laryngoscope blade at the right corner of the patient's mouth and sweep the tongue to the left while advancing the blade posteriorly along the palate.

f. Extend the left arm forward at the shoulder in order to lift the patient's tongue and jaw.

g. Position yourself so that your line of vision follows the line of the laryngoscope blade.

h. If the anatomy is obscured by secretions, use suction to clear the airway.

i. It the glottic opening is not visualized within 15 seconds, remove the laryngoscope and ventilate the patient by bag-valve-mask prior to reattempting visualization.

Note: Hold the laryngoscope in the left hand, regardless of which hand is dominant.

Note: Advance the tip of a straight blade posterior to the epiglottis so that the tip of the blade lifts the epiglottis from the glottic opening.

The tip of a curved blade should come to rest in the vallecula, just superior to the epiglottis.

Note: The line of force should be at a 45° angle to the patient's face. Do not rotate your forearm or hand, as this causes the patient's teeth to become the fulcrum of a lever (the laryngoscope blade). This may result in trauma and will not likely facilitate visualization.

Note: Assuming a position directly above the patient's head usually does not afford a view of the glottis. It is best to assume a position slightly behind the patient's head.

Task Analysis (*continued*)

Primary Step	Subcomponents	Notes
10. Place the endotracheal tube.	**a.** Hold the endotracheal tube in your right hand with a pencil grip, just below the adapter for the ventilation device.	*Note:* The tip of the tube must be curved upward to facilitate passage through the glottis.
	b. Advance the tube into the patient's mouth and direct it inferiorly toward the glottic opening.	The tube may have to be directed slightly anteriorly. The use of stylet or a Trigger® Tube (Mallinckrodt Medical) may be useful to achieve this anterior direction.
	c. Advance the tip of the tube between the vocal cords until the cuff has passed approximately 5 mm beyond the cords.	
	d. If the tube has not been placed within 30 seconds of interrupting ventilations, stop and reventilate the patient prior to making another attempt to intubate.	Maintain manual stabilization of the tube until correct positioning has been assured and the tube has been secured using tape or a commercially made device.
	e. Manually stabilize the tube in this position with your right hand while carefully withdrawing the laryngoscope and lying it aside.	
	f. Use your left hand to depress the plunger of the syringe to inflate the cuff of the endotracheal tube.	*Note:* Keep the plunger of the syringe depressed until it is disconnected from the inflation port. The inflation port has a valve that will allow air to escape the cuff when the tip of the syringe is secured in the port.
	g. Disconnect the syringe from the inflation port.	Keep the syringe easily available in the event that the cuff must be deflated to reposition the tube.

142

11. Verify correct placement of the tube.

a. Instruct an assistant to remove the mask from the bag-valve device and attach the adapter to the endotracheal tube.

b. Position the diaphragm of your stethoscope on the patient's right anterior chest.

c. Instruct the assistant to ventilate the patient as you auscultate the right chest for breath sounds.

d. Instruct the assistant to ventilate the patient as you auscultate the left chest.

e. Instruct the assistant to ventilate the patient as you auscultate over the epigastrium.

f. Once correct placement is confirmed, instruct the assistant to ventilate the patient.

Note: Visualizing the tube pass through the glottis and hearing breath sounds are definitive indicators of endotracheal placement of the tube.

Absence of breath sounds bilaterally upon ventilation and positive insufflation of the stomach indicates esophageal placement of the tube. If this occurs, **THE ENDOTRACHEAL TUBE MUST BE REMOVED IMMEDIATELY AND THE PATIENT MUST BE VENTILATED BY BAG-VALVE-MASK PRIOR TO REATTEMPTING INTUBATION.**

To remove the endotracheal tube, turn the patient's head to the side (or, if feasible, turn the patient onto his or her left side), use the syringe to deflate the cuff of the tube and smoothly withdraw the endotracheal tube. Be prepared to suction, because this action often precipitates regurgitation.

If placement of the endotracheal tube is in question or if required by local protocol, adjunctive devices to check placement are available (e.g., end-tidal CO_2 detection and aspiration devices).

Task Analysis (continued)

Primary Step	Subcomponents	Notes
12. Secure the endotracheal tube.	**a.** Continue manual stabilization of the endotracheal tube. **b.** Either tape or a commercially manufactured device may be used to secure the tube. **c.** One method for securing the tube with tape is as follows: • Tear a piece of 2-in.-wide tape that is approximately 3 in. longer that the circumference of the patient's head. • Fold the middle third of the tape in half lengthwise, so that it sticks to itself. • Place the folded portion of the tape under the patient's head, with the exposed	Breath sounds present on the right side but absent on the left indicate probable right main stem bronchus placement of the tip of the tube. In this case, the cuff should be deflated and the tube very slightly withdrawn until bilateral breath sounds are auscultated. The cuff is then reinflated. *Note:* A qualified assistant may stabilize the tube as you prepare to secure it or may prepare to secure the tube as you manually stabilize it. Tape has the disadvantage of not securely holding the tube if the patient's skin is moist. The use of tincture of benzoin or a similar product may enhance the adhesion of the tape. If tape is used, there are a variety of configurations that may be used.

adhesive at the ends facing upward.

- Take one end of the tape and make a lengthwise tear approximately 1½ in. into it.
- Pull this end of the tape across the patient's face, toward the tube.
- Wrap the split ends of the tape in opposite directions around the tube.
- Repeat with the opposite end of the tape, pulling it securely against the patient's head and face before wrapping the ends around the tube.
- Make a note of the depth marking (in centimeters) at the point where the tube enters the patient's mouth.

Rationale: To establish a point of reference to determine if the depth of the tube has changed during ventilation or while moving the patient.

- Stabilize the patient's head and neck when moving the patient.

Rationale: Hyperextension of the neck may cause the tube to become dislodged from the trachea.

145

Training Needs Analysis

A **needs analysis** is a study of the existing level of employee performance compared to stated or desired levels of performance, such as institutional or industry standards (Donaldson and Scannell 1986). Ideally, performance data should be collected in a systemwide CQI program. The difference between the current and the desired performance is called a **performance gap.** The goal of training is to close the performance gap. It is essential to remember, though, that not all performance gaps are a result of deficient knowledge or skills. For example, an ALS response goal of 8 minutes or less 90% of the time depends very little on training, unless knowledge of area geography is an issue. Meeting this goal depends much more on efficient dispatching and strategic vehicle location. The human factors involved, such as slow response to dispatched information, are generally not due to a lack of knowledge of *how* to make it to the vehicle and mark responding, but instead are generally affective issues.

Needs analysis on an individual level should be part of employee hiring and orientation and can be conducted through performance testing, protocol tests, and observation by field training officers with the assistance of an orientation checklist. Institutional or agency continuing education should be based on CQI audits of critical skills to identify the need for training in airway management, recognition of critical trauma patients, compliance with protocols, and other performance areas. Needs analysis can also be conducted by keeping abreast of industry trends and emerging standards.

In addition to the preceding, a needs analysis must consider how the outcomes of training will be evaluated. Training programs can be costly and management or external clients will want to know if they have effectively spent their money. Finally, your needs analysis should result in the preparation of a **training proposal** or plan through which you will communicate your findings and recommendations to decision makers. Box 9-3 lists the critical parts of a training proposal, and Box 9-4 gives a sample training proposal.

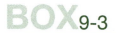

BOX 9-3

Components of a Training Proposal

- What is the objective of the training?
- What is the need for training, and how was the need identified and measured?
- Who needs the training?
- What is the expected outcome of the training?
- How will the outcomes be measured?
- What resources are required?
- When should the training take place?
- How will the training benefit the individual and the organization?
- What is the likely outcome *without* training?
- What is the cost of the training?
  - Instructional development time
  - Overtime for attendees
  - Clerical expenses
  - Speaker expenses
  - Facility and equipment expenses
- What are the sample training syllabus and schedule?

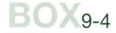

BOX 9-4

Sample Training Proposal

Training Proposal for City Ambulance Service

Prepared by R. Smith Associates
February 27, 2004

TRAINING OBJECTIVE:	To prepare all Ambulance Service ALS personnel to perform rapid sequence induction of anesthesia (RSI) for endotracheal intubation of the responsive patient in need of immediate airway control.
NEED FOR TRAINING:	Concerns expressed by area emergency department physicians and ambulance service paramedics about several critical incidents involving the inability to secure an airway on

responsive patients in need of intubation prompted a patient care report audit on Code 1 ALS transports for the past 12 months. The audit determined that in this period of time there were 21 adult trauma and 15 adult medical patients who arrived at the ED without definitive airway control and effective ventilation who would have been candidates for RSI using the protocol established by the medical control committee for Clark County.

EXPECTED RESULTS: Training is expected to result in a 95% intubation success rate for responsive patients with the use of RSI.

TARGET AUDIENCE: All nonprobationary paramedic employees.

EVALUATION: Patient care reports for all adult patients in whom RSI was indicated, whether successfully performed or not, will be audited for 6 months following training.

RESOURCES NEEDED: Classroom space, cooperation of anesthesia for clinical rotations.

TIME FRAME: Training should commence immediately upon approval of the proposal.

BENEFITS: The primary benefits to individual employees and the organization include enhanced success in the performance of a critical skill.

EXPECTED OUTCOME WITHOUT PROGRAM: Without this training program, it is quite possible that the organization and individual providers will be placed at greater risk for professional liability for failed airway maintenance, particularly since RSI is a standard of practice in 90% of the ALS agencies in the state.

PROGRAM COST: The costs of this program are negligible, because it will rely on current EMS education staff and the existing on-duty in-service schedule.

NOTE: *A sample syllabus and schedule are included as attachments to a training proposal.*

NOTE: *There are a number of considerations in determining and communicating program costs that are beyond the scope of this text.*

Summary

Systematic planning is essential to ensuring that educational programs are needed and that their content meets the needs of learners and stakeholders. Job analysis and needs analysis are indispensable tools for determining the competencies, needs, and tasks of a job, and task analysis is critical in deconstructing tasks to their elemental parts in order to effectively plan for teaching them. Finally, these findings and recommendations need to be communicated to decision makers in such a way that the need for and benefits of training and education programs are clear. An organized, concise training proposal communicates this information nicely.

REVIEW QUESTIONS

1. Describe the process of job analysis.

2. Explain the importance of performing task analyses.

3. What is the goal of educational needs analysis?

4. What type of information is communicated in a training proposal?

Developing Instructional Objectives

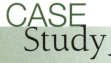

CASE Study

Danny Torres is the EMS liaison for St. Luke's Hospital. The emergency department is sponsoring a continuing education series for EMS providers and Danny is getting ready to write the objectives for a 4-hour session on poisoning. It seems that several students from the local college have been transported to St. Luke's recently suffering from acute alcohol poisoning and the use of a variety of illegal substances. A recent survey of EMS personnel that transport to St. Luke's revealed that many of the providers were unsure how to recognize the signs and symptoms associated with the use of these drugs and weren't sure if their treatment was as good as it could be in these cases.

Questions

1. Where should Danny begin the process of writing objectives for this program?
2. What uses of the objectives should Danny keep in mind as he writes them?
3. What question can Danny ask himself that will help him formulate objectives to meet the needs of the attendees?

Introduction

Previous chapters have alluded to the importance of developing effective instructional objectives, and Chapters 7, 8, and 9 laid important groundwork for the process of developing instructional objectives. Instructional objectives stem from the competencies noted in a job analysis and are identified through cognitive and psychomotor task analyses. Objectives serve as the basis of lesson planning, selection of teaching-learning methods, and evaluation. As the NSC are replaced with educational standards, we will no longer see the detailed objectives contained in current NSC documents. Although writing and using effective instructional objectives have always been important skills for educators, they will become even more critical as we move into the future.

KEY TERMS

competency, p. 153

goal, p. 153

terminal performance
objective, p. 153

enabling objective, p. 153

proxy, p. 159

Goals, Competencies, and Objectives

There are important distinctions between goals and objectives in the context of education. **Goals** are very broad statements of what an educational program or course intends to accomplish. For example, the goal

goal
A broad statement of the intended outcomes of the program.

A goal is a broad statement of the intended outcomes of the educational program.

competency
A statement describing a primary task of a job.

terminal performance objective
A competency.

enabling objective
A lower-level objective whose performance is necessary to achieve a competency.

Competencies are also known as terminal performance objectives. Competencies are statements of the primary tasks of a job.

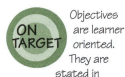

Objectives are learner oriented. They are stated in terms of what the learner is expected to do.

of a paramedic program may be to prepare students for entry-level paramedic positions in the prehospital-care setting. This is a statement of the final outcome and is oriented toward what the *program* is to accomplish.

Competencies, also known as **terminal performance objectives** (TPOs), are the primary tasks of a job. Competencies are statements of what students need to accomplish in order for the program to meet its goal. Ideally, competencies include a statement of the circumstances of performance (conditions) and the degree of accuracy or proficiency required (criterion). An example is: The student should be able to perform endotracheal intubation in the patient in respiratory failure or respiratory arrest in the prehospital setting with less than 30 seconds interruption in patient ventilation. The conditions of performance are "in the patient in respiratory failure or arrest" and "in the prehospital setting." The proficiency criterion is "with less than 30 seconds interruption in patient ventilation." This is a major advanced life-support skill that can, and must, be broken down into its component parts for teaching and learning activities. Goals and objectives are structured hierarchically, with lower-level **(enabling) objectives** cascading from the goals and TPOs. The TPO serves as a major category of performance under which lower-level enabling objectives are developed. TPOs are complex and may implicitly involve behaviors in all three domains of learning.

Objectives are statements of expected behaviors, knowledge, and attitudes necessary to the attainment of competencies. Objectives are phrased using verbs that allow for measurement of educational attainment and are *learner oriented*. Objectives are always written in terms of what we expect the *student* or *learner* to do. The verbs used to describe expected performance are precise and measurable. Objectives fall into one of the three domains of learning and vary in levels of complexity. (Refer to Tables 7-1, 7-2, and 7-3 for a review of the three domains of learning, the levels of learning within each domain, and examples of verbs used at each level.)

Objectives are generally listed under a common stem statement such as, "At the end of this lesson the learner (or participant) should be able to." Some sources recommend the stem, "The student *will* be able to." However, as educators we can only set the conditions that make it likely that a student will learn; we cannot guarantee student learning. Learning is ultimately the student's activity. In this litigious society, educators should use caution that they are not implying a guarantee of student learning that puts the onus of student failure on the shoulders of the educator.

It is important to note that many people will refer to instructional objectives as *behavioral objectives*. Indeed, we are interested in behaviors and rely on observed behaviors as evidence of learning. The term behavioral objective can be a bit limiting, in that not all learning is as directly observable as the term behavioral implies. In our quest for directly measurable attributes, we must take care that we don't adopt the view that if it can't be measured, it doesn't exist. Learning is far too complex for us to be able to measure all aspects of it precisely. Certainly measurement is important, but we shouldn't allow obsession with measurement to restrict teaching and learning to only those activities that we can directly and objectively measure. Nonetheless, we rightfully exist in a competency-based field and must strive to measure critical aspects of performance.

From Competency to Objectives

We will assume that we are working in an educational program with a prespecified goal of creating competent entry-level EMS personnel. We begin with competencies as the basis for writing instructional objectives, assuming that a job analysis has revealed required competencies.

Example 1

We begin with the following competency, or TPO:

- **The student should be able to formulate a prehospital treatment plan for the patient with suspected acute coronary syndrome.**

The conditions of "prehospital" and "patient with suspected acute coronary syndrome" are specified. There is not a proficiency or accuracy criterion here because we know that, given the limited amount of diagnostic information available in the prehospital setting, it would be unrealistic to expect 100% accuracy, and any other number assigned would be arbitrary. Ideally, we would have an industry standard, based on research, to guide us in determining the proficiency level.

We must analyze this competency by breaking it down into the component cognitive and psychomotor objectives, the performance of which will result in accomplishment of the competency. First, it is obvious that the learner must recognize a patient with suspected acute coronary syndrome. This is a high-level behavior that relies on yet many more lower-level activities. We can write an objective for this behavior as follows:

- **The student should be able to formulate a field impression of acute coronary syndrome (ACS) when presented with a patient who has signs, symptoms, and history consistent with ACS.**

Recalling the domains and levels of learning, the act of *formulating* is a cognitive behavior at the synthesis level. In the current NSC, this would be considered a Level 3, or problem-solving, objective. Being a high-level objective, several lower-level objectives are prerequisite to its attainment. What knowledge and skills are necessary to formulating a field impression for ACS? Consider the following:

- **The student should be able to differentiate between the signs and symptoms of, and history consistent with, ACS and those of clinical presentations that may be confused with ACS.**

This is a cognitive objective at the *analysis* level. The student must distinguish between the overall presentation of ACS and that of other emergencies, such as pulmonary embolism. The learner is breaking apart the big picture and looking for patterns that fit with existing schemata. In order to do this, the student must have some idea of what the information with which he or she is working means.

- **The student should be able to recognize the signs, symptoms, and historical factors consistent with ACS.**

This is a cognitive objective at the application level. Although *recognize* could be used at the knowledge level, the behavior of interest is that, when presented with a patient who has signs and symptoms, the learner will *apply* his or her knowledge of what the signs and symptoms are to a new situation. Essentially, the student's conscious or unconscious mental process is to compare what he or she finds out about the patient to the schema for ACS—and perhaps the schemata for some related disorders—and determine whether or not this patient's signs and symptoms are consistent with ACS. We now must consider what condition or conditions are prerequisite to recognition.

- **The student should be able to list the signs, symptoms, and historical factors indicative of ACS.**

This is a cognitive objective at the knowledge level. Simply put, the learner must know what the signs and symptoms of ACS are before he or she can recognize them in a situation.

- **The student should be able to perform a physical examination.**

This is a psychomotor objective at the level of complex, overt response. In order to find the signs of ACS, the student must be able to elicit them during a physical examination. At this point, this particular objective would probably have been included in an earlier lesson on physical examination and would not be repeated in a lesson on treating ACS. This illustrates the importance of appropriately sequencing instruction.

If we were to continue, these objectives would branch in different directions and eventually take us back to objectives appropriate to the EMT-Basic level.

- **The student should be able to obtain a blood pressure by auscultation.**

This is a psychomotor objective at the mechanism level. Beyond this level, the steps of obtaining a blood pressure by auscultation would be included in a task analysis that would become part of the lesson plan content supporting this objective.

Obviously this example is for illustrative purposes and does not go through the entire process of developing all the objectives necessary for a curriculum or even a module or lesson. But take this opportunity to consider what other objectives—psychomotor, cognitive, and affective—are related to the given competency and higher-level objectives.

Example 2

In this example, we begin with the following competency, or TPO:

- **The student should be able to manage the out-of-hospital cardiac arrest patient.**

Again, we have a statement indicating under what conditions the student is expected to perform, but we do not have an industry standard to guide us in specifying a proficiency criterion. In the previous example we considered the formulation of a treatment plan, which did not include implementation of the plan. In this example we are working with a much more broadly stated competency, in which we need to consider not only the formulation of a treatment plan and recognition of the patient's condition, but also the skills involved in implementing the plan, directing team members, considering transport and field termination of resuscitation options, ongoing assessment of the patient, and revision of the treatment plan.

Once again, this is an illustrative example and as such we do not carry it out to completion, but we can use it to explore possibilities. We can use the following objective as a starting point:

- **The student should be able to evaluate the appropriateness of considering field termination of resuscitative efforts.**

What knowledge, values, and skills must the learner have in order to do this? Consider the following:

- **The student should be able to interpret applicable local and state laws and regulations as they apply to a given cardiac arrest scenario.**

In order to do this, the student would have to comprehend the laws and would have to compare the particulars of a given situation to the laws and regulations. This would involve complex behaviors such as analysis of the current situation and evaluation of the current situation against the criteria of the laws and regulations. How could you write such objectives?

- **The student should be able to empathize with the family of the cardiac arrest patient when considering management options.**

This is an affective objective at the organization level. It requires not only lower-level affective abilities, but knowledge of the situation as well.

- **The student must be able to explain the pathophysiological process of cardiac arrest.**

This is a cognitive objective at the comprehension level. Because we can't directly see student understanding, we rely on his or her explanation of pathophysiology to demonstrate understanding. Without an understanding of the pathophysiological process of cardiac arrest, the student will be unable to determine whether attempted or continued resuscitation is appropriate or not. Without this information, the student will not be able to give the family the appropriate information.

Objectives as the Basis for Lesson Planning and Selection of Teaching-Learning Activities

Objectives are used to build lesson plans and to select appropriate teaching-learning activities. The objectives are stated at the beginning of the lesson plan and must be conveyed to the learners. Not only must we make the desired learning outcomes available to students, but we must also make sure students understand how they should be using the objectives.

Students often see objectives only as a guide to the lesson content, unaware that the verb used in the objective tells them in what way they will be expected to use the content. For example, a student may be given an objective such as: At the end of this lesson you should be able to recognize the patient having an allergic reaction. Students often see this in terms of a multiple choice question asking, Which of the following is a sign of an allergic reaction? However, the objective implies that in the clinical setting, or given a scenario, the student will be able to recognize a patient who is having an allergic reaction. This means that the student will have to know what signs, symptoms, and historical information are indicative of an allergic reaction *and* that the student must recognize them when he or she actually encounters them, not when he or she is presented with a list of signs and symptoms from which to pick and choose.

PEARLS Students must know how they are expected to use the objectives. They often only see them as a guide to course content, not as an indication of what they should be able to do. Discuss the use of objectives with your students, rather than just telling them what the objectives are.

Not only is it necessary to clarify the meaning of objectives with students, but we must use this same information to decide what to put in the lesson plan, how to present it, and what activities in and out of class will support the learning outcomes we actually desire. Going back to the objective in the previous paragraph, it is easy to see that listing the signs and symptoms and causes of allergic reactions is only preliminary, background learning. This information must be reinforced with case studies and scenarios in which the student has to apply the knowledge. A scenario or case study should not tell the students what the signs and symptoms are but should present them in the way they would be encountered in real life. For example, the case study should not state, The patient is hypotensive and has hives. We rarely encounter a patient who says this or is tattooed with the information "I'm hypotensive" or "These are hives." In this case, the student is not *recognizing* the signs and symptoms; they are being *given* to him. Consider instead, giving a case study description that states, The patient is complaining of feeling faint and you notice red blotches on his skin.

It is critical to state the objective using a verb that describes the behavior you really want the learner to perform.

As a corollary to recognizing an allergic reaction, the student must also recognize what is not an allergic reaction. It is important, too, that you present scenarios or case studies in which the patient complains of something such as being stung by a wasp or even in which the patient says he or she is having an allergic reaction, but in which the signs and symptoms do not represent an allergic reaction. A helpful homework

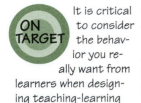

problem would be to present a scenario and ask students to determine whether or not the patient is having an allergic reaction and to justify their answers by explaining why or why not. It is not particularly effective to offer homework problems such as, "A patient who has been stung by a bee and who has difficulty breathing, hypotension, and hives may be suffering from a/an _____ reaction." This type of problem does not get at the higher-level cognitive functions, in this case, recognition, for which we are looking from our students.

Objectives as the Basis for Evaluation

Because it is the attainment of objectives in which we are interested, we must have a way of measuring students' performance against the criteria set forth by the objectives. Again, objectives are not simply a guide to the content of a quiz, exam, homework assignment, skills checklist, or clinical evaluation form. The items on these evaluations must ask the student to perform the same activity required by the objective. This requires that objectives be thoughtfully prepared in program planning and that the item writer consider the intent of the objective. Realistically, we cannot always measure performance under real-life conditions. In this case, we must make sure that the knowledge and behaviors we are asking students to demonstrate are representative of the true behaviors of interest. In this sense, an exam serves as a **proxy**, or surrogate, for the conditions of performance we actually desire.

proxy
A substitute or alternate.

Example 1

Suppose that one of our objectives is as follows:

- **Given a scenario, the student should be able to identify whether or not a patient meets trauma triage criteria for transportation to a trauma center.**

The first thing the objective tells us is that the student must perform the desired behavior in the context of a scenario. This particular objective could be measured in the clinical setting, laboratory, or on a written examination. Usually, the difficulty is in translating the objective into an effective written item rather than observing performance in a lab or clinical setting. You will learn much more about different types of exam items later in the text, but for now we assume that we are writing a multiple-choice item.

In the preceding objective, we are asking the student to identify whether or not a particular patient meets criteria for transportation to a trauma center. We cannot tell if the student is able to identify the criteria in a patient if we ask a question such as this:

- Which of the following is a trauma triage criterion for transport to a trauma center?
  a. Fall from a height greater than three times the height of the patient.
  b. Receiving an injury while under the influence of alcohol or narcotics.
  c. Penetrating trauma to a distal extremity.
  d. Being involved in a motor vehicle collision.

The most we can tell about a student who answers this correctly (assuming he or she did not guess the answer) is that the student can pick the most likely of four choices from a list. It does not tell us whether or not the student would recognize that criterion, or any other, in context. The following multiple-choice item is a better surrogate for what we want the student to be able to do, based on the objective:

- You have arrived on the scene of a vehicle collision with four patients. Which of the following patients meets trauma triage criteria for transport to a trauma center?
  a. A 52-year-old male was the restrained driver of vehicle 1, which sustained 10 inches of deformity to the front end of the automobile. He has a GCS of 15 and is complaining of pain in his left shoulder.
  b. A 47-year-old woman was the unrestrained front-seat passenger in vehicle 1. She has deformity of her nose with evidence of moderate bleeding that was controlled upon your arrival. She has a GCS of 15, a blood pressure of 110/78, and a heart rate of 92.
  c. A 22-year-old male was the driver of vehicle 2. Vehicle 2 has 15 inches of interior compartment intrusion on the driver's side, and the driver is unresponsive, apneic, pulseless, and has a nearly complete decapitating injury.
  d. A 21-year-old female was the restrained front-seat passenger of vehicle 2. She is alert with a GCS of 15, is complaining of neck and left shoulder pain, and has a blood pressure of 112/80 and a respiratory rate of 24.

Example 2

Begin with the following objective:

- **The student should be able to evaluate the appropriateness of a treatment plan for the patient in hypovolemic shock.**

Evaluation is a high-level cognitive objective in which the student is expected to judge the value of something against given criteria. Therefore, a test item should ask the student to consider treatment plans and decide on their value for the patient in hypovolemic shock. This calls for more than recognizing a single appropriate measure. It also requires the student to consider the sequence of interventions.

- **Your patient is a 37-year-old male who has been stabbed in the groin and has lost approximately 2 liters of blood. He is pale and diaphoretic, is confused and agitated, and has a heart rate of 124 and a blood pressure of 72/50. Which of the following treatment plans is most appropriate?**
  - a. **Immediately control any ongoing bleeding, apply a nonrebreather mask with oxygen at 15 L/min, immobilize the cervical spine, and transport.**
  - b. **Apply a nonrebreather mask with oxygen at 15 L/min, control ongoing bleeding, initiate two large-bore lines of crystalloid solution enroute to the trauma center, and monitor the patient for signs of improved perfusion.**
  - c. **Ventilate the patient with a bag-valve-mask device using supplemental oxygen, start two large-bore IVs of crystalloid solution, apply pressure to the femoral artery, transport, and monitor the patient for changes.**
  - d. **Place an oropharyngeal airway, ventilate the patient using supplemental oxygen, place a cervical collar on the patient, use direct pressure to control bleeding, immobilize the patient on a long back board, and intubate the patient enroute to the trauma center.**

Summary

Valuing the need for construction of sound objectives requires the ability to see the "big picture" of the other educational functions that rely upon these objectives. Writing instructional objectives is an essential educational function and is a skill that takes time and plenty of feedback to acquire. Objectives must be worded to reflect what it is we really want students to be able to do in order to guide us appropriately in constructing lesson plans, teaching-learning activities, and assessments. In the future, as we move away from prescriptive NSC, the ability to write effective objectives will be paramount to the success of the EMS education endeavor.

REVIEW QUESTIONS

1. What is the relationship between goals, competencies, and objectives?

2. What role do objectives play in creating a lesson plan?

3. What role do objectives play in assessment?

4. Why is the wording of objectives critical?

5. What are the components of a competency?

Packaging
the Program

Learning Objectives

Upon completion of this chapter you should be able to

- Discuss considerations in assigning credit hours to classroom, laboratory, and clinical courses.

- Consider various formats for delivering EMT-B, EMT-I, and EMT-P programs using a semester-based format.

- Consider various formats for delivering EMT-B, EMT-I, and EMT-P programs using a modular approach.

- Discuss considerations in obtaining approval for CEUs for EMS programs and courses.

- Create a course or program syllabus.

CASE
Study

Barbara Williams-White has been a secondary instructor for 3 years and has just been hired as a primary instructor in the EMS program at Graves Community College. The EMS program department chair, Janie Brown, has asked Barbara to take a look at the current EMT-Basic program format and to come up with ideas for revising the course. The course is currently one semester long, with a 5-credit-hour lecture, a 1-credit-hour laboratory, and a 1-credit-hour clinical course.

Questions

1. What questions should Barbara ask before she begins her work?

2. What other program formats might be recommended?

3. If the length of the course changes, how does this affect the number of credit hours?

4. What boundaries will Barbara need to consider?

Introduction

There are several considerations in packaging the contents of a course or program that will vary depending upon the context in which you work as an EMS educator. In this chapter we consider the assignment of credit hours, distributing course work using a semester-based or modular format, obtaining CEUs for continuing education offerings, and creating a course syllabus. Attention to the distribution of course work is important, as the syllabus usually serves as the basis for course approval by state regulatory agencies.

Credit Hours and Semesters

Conventionally, credit hours are assigned to course work in community colleges and universities using a given ratio of clock hours to credit hours. It should be noted that the instructional hour is often considered to be 50 minutes.

- Didactic (lecture/classroom) courses: 1 clock hour per week = 1 credit hour per semester.
- Laboratory courses: 2 clock hours per week = 1 credit hour per semester.
- Clinical courses: 3 clock hours per week = 1 credit hour per semester.

This lends itself to a variety of formats for part-time and full-time programs, based on a 16-week semester (15 instructional weeks, 1 final-exam week).

PEARLS Some academic institutions operate on quarters rather than semesters.

Example 1: Two-Semester EMT-Basic Course

Although the EMT-B (EMT-Basic) NSC is a 110-hour curriculum (**http://www.nhtsa.dot.gov/people/injury/ems/pub/emtbnsc.pdf**), many universities and community colleges offer courses that are approximately

200 hours in length. Remember that the EMT-B NSC requirement of 110 hours can be considered a minimum. However, also keep in mind that some states have restrictions on the maximum number of hours for EMS courses. Following is one example of how a two-semester course could look.

SEMESTER 1

- EMT-Basic Lecture I
  - Meets twice per week for 2 hours.
  - 4 clock hours per week = 4 credit hours per semester.
  - 15 weeks $\times$ 4 hours = 60 clock hours.

- EMT-Basic Lab I
  - Meets once per week for 2 hours.
  - 2 clock hours per week = 1 credit hour per semester.
  - 15 weeks $\times$ 2 hours = 30 clock hours.

- EMT-Basic Clinical I
  - Students attend 40 hours of field and emergency department clinical rotations for 1 credit hour (even though this is less than the recommended ratio of clock hours to credit hours for clinical courses, it is not possible to assign less than 1 credit hour in most cases).

Total: 90 hours of lecture and lab, 6 credit hours

SEMESTER 2

- EMT-Basic Lecture II
  - Meets once per week for 2 hours.
  - 2 clock hours per week = 2 credit hours per semester.
  - 15 weeks $\times$ 2 hours = 30 clock hours.

- EMT-Basic Lab II
  - Meets once per week for 4 hours.
  - 4 clock hours per week = 2 credit hours per semester.
  - 15 weeks $\times$ 4 hours = 60 clock hours.

- EMT-Basic Clinical II
  - Students attend 40 hours of field and emergency department clinical rotations for 1 credit hour.

Total: 90 hours of lecture and lab, 5 credit hours
Two-Semester Total: 180 hours of lecture and lab, 11 credit hours

A configuration such as this, with 180 hours of lecture and laboratory time and ample clinical opportunities, makes it possible for EMT-Basics to be entry-level competent, requiring a minimum of on-the-job training following certification. In addition, with quality instruction, students are better prepared for the demands of the EMT-Intermediate or EMT-Paramedic curriculum.

Example 2: One-Semester EMT-Basic Course

- Lecture meets for 2.5 hours twice per week.
  - 5 clock hours per week = 5 credit hours per semester.
  - 5 clock hours per week × 15 weeks = 75 clock hours per semester.
- Lab meets for 4 hours once per week.
  - 4 clock hours per week = 2 credit hours per semester.
  - 4 clock hours per week × 15 weeks = 60 clock hours.
- Students attend clinical hours as determined by the program.

  Total: 135 hours of lecture and lab, 7 credit hours

Example 3: Two-Semester Paramedic Program (Full-Time)

Note that a full credit load is generally between 12 and 18 credit hours per semester.

SEMESTER 1

- Lecture meets for two 5-hour days per week.
  - 10 clock hours per week = 10 credit hours per semester.
  - 10 clock hours × 15 weeks = 150 hours of lecture.
- Lab meets for one 4-hour session per week.
  - 4 clock hours per week = 2 credit hours per semester.
  - 4 clock hours × 15 weeks = 60 hours of lab.
- Students attend clinical (on the average) 16 hours per week.
  - 16 clock hours per week = 5 credit hours per semester (rounded down from 5.3).
  - 16 clock hours × 15 weeks = 240 hours of clinical.

SEMESTER 2

- Lecture meets for two 5-hour days per week.
  - 10 clock hours per week = 10 credit hours per semester.
  - 10 clock hours × 15 weeks = 150 hours of lecture.

- Lab meets for one 2-hour session per week.
  - 2 clock hours per week = 1 credit hour per semester.
  - 2 clock hours per week × 15 weeks = 30 hours of lab.
- Students attend clinical (on the average) 8 hours per week.
  - 8 clock hours per week = 3 credit hours per semester (rounded up from 2.6).
  - 8 clock hours per week × 15 weeks = 120 hours of clinical.
- Students attend field internship (on the average) 8 hours per week.
  - 8 clock hours per week = 2 credit hours per semester (rounded down from 2.6).
  - 8 clock hours per week × 15 weeks = 120 hours of internship.

> **Program Total:** **300 hours of lecture**
> **90 hours of lab**
> **360 hours of clinical**
> **120 hours of field internship**
> **= 870 program hours**

The total of 870 hours is shorter than average for a paramedic program. There are often difficult choices to make when trying to fit a program into an academic setting, rather than creating a program *for* an academic setting. Semester length may not correlate with state requirements for program length. At other times, a competing program may make its course more attractive to employers by creating a compact course. If the employer is paying employees to attend and paying overtime to fulfill the employees' work obligations, shorter is more attractive. Beyond a certain amount of compression, though, quality of teaching suffers and students cannot keep up with reading, studying, course assignments, and clinical rotations. On the other hand, there is no evidence that a longer-than-average course results in better outcomes. Most paramedic courses are between 1000 and 1500 hours, including didactic, lab, and clinical.

PEARLS Although the shorter program may increase enrollment in the short term, if the quality of the program has been compromised, its reputation will soon suffer.

Modular Formats

Programs offered by hospitals, fire departments, or other nonacademic settings often use a modular approach to packaging their programs, based on the NSC modules. The lengths of the courses are not restricted to a semester schedule and continue until the program has met the desired number of hours. Courses are generally offered in part-time formats, meeting 3 or 4 hours twice per week, plus clinical rotations; or in an academy-style format, meeting 8 hours per day, 40 hours per week with clinical either interspersed with lecture and lab or following the lecture and lab components.

The NSC list recommended ranges of hours for the curricula to assist in establishing the time frame, and thus the number of class sessions, for each module and can be found at **http://www.nhtsa. dot.gov/ people/injury/ems/nsc.htm#emt**.

Packaging Continuing Education Courses

Most states have a one-to-one ratio of clock hours to continuing education credits or units (CECs or CEUs). Generally, there are required topics and "other" categories. Usually there is a compulsory minimum number of hours for the required topics and a maximum number of hours allowed in other areas. You need to refer to the guidelines of your state EMS office for the approval of continuing education programs. You can find a detailed explanation of the Continuing Education Coordinating Board for EMS (CECBEMS) requirements for course approval on its website at **http://www.cecbems.org /forms/ app-explain.doc**.

Creating a Course Syllabus

The purpose of a course syllabus is to provide a description of the course, its goals, student objectives, policies and procedures, grading and examination requirements, required textbooks, instructor contact information, and a course schedule. Some institutions have standard formats for course syllabi, whereas others consider the format of the syllabus to be at the instructor's discretion. A sample course syllabus is provided in Box 11-1 for your reference.

Sample Course Schedule

Refer to Figure 11-1 for an example of a course schedule, which is part of the syllabus for classes with a regular meeting schedule.

Box11-1

EMS 250—Paramedic Clinical Rotation I Fall 2003

Credit: 3

Time and Location: By arrangement

Course Description: EMS 250 provides students the opportunity for participation in patient care activities in various hospital and field clinical settings. Students are expected to integrate knowledge and skills into professional practice. Activities during clinical rotations are closely supervised and guided by clinical preceptors. Learning is evaluated in a variety of ways to assess student progress toward the course and, ultimately, program goals. The goals of this course are that students: (1) Develop advanced life support skills, such as EKG interpretation and medication administration, (2) augment basic life support skills, (3) formulate and implement treatment plans, and (4) serve as the team leader for basic life-support calls.

Course Instructor: J. Phillips, Associate Professor of EMS
240 Pierce Hall
1803 University Drive
(212) 555-0000
e-mail: jrp@university.edu
Office hours: By appointment

Prerequisites: All students must be currently certified in CPR for health-care providers and as EMT-Basics in order to participate in clinical experiences. These certifications must be maintained throughout the program. Lapsed certifications will result in the suspension of the student's clinical attendance privileges until the certifications are renewed and on file with the program. Any absences as a result of lapsed certification will be considered unexcused. Additionally, students must have completed and filed with Student Health Services the required student health record documenting immunization prior to attending clinical rotations. Students must also have filed with the program a criminal history check as required in the program *Clinical Handbook*.

Course Objectives: At the completion of this course the student should be able to demonstrate satisfactory progress toward the program goal of becoming a competent entry-level paramedic by

01.   Demonstrating patient care interventions learned in EMS 240.
02.   Developing work organization skills.
03.   Adopting professional characteristics and behaviors.
04.   Developing critical thinking and problem-solving skills.

05. Integrating patient assessment information with knowledge of pathophysiology to formulate field impressions of patient problems.
06. Developing patient treatment plans.
07. Modifying the treatment plan based on continuous evaluation of its effectiveness.

Required Text: All students are required to purchase a FISDAP® account online through the FISDAP® Web site at **www.FISDAP.net**. FISDAP® is an interactive Web-based program for scheduling and documentation of student clinical experiences.

Teaching Methods: In order to arrange the conditions most favorable to student learning, this course relies on guidance of and reflection on student experiences. Assignments, as well as interactions with preceptors and the course instructor (clinical coordinator), are structured to guide student's thinking and reflection on his or her experiences.

Evaluation Methods: Achievement of the course goals and their related objectives will be assessed using preceptor observations, documentation of clinical activities, student assignments, patient care documentation, and short, directed journaling activities. Students will be assessed for their ability to demonstrate skills, knowledge, and professional attributes. Point values will be assigned to the evaluation process, and the student will receive a letter grade for the course.

Course Policies: In addition to the information contained in this syllabus, students are held to the guidelines in the EMS Program's *Clinical Handbook and Resource Packet*. The resource addresses policies and guidelines that apply to all intermediate and paramedic clinical courses and the field internship. Students are also responsible for any announcements or policy revisions distributed.

Clinical Hours and Activities: In order to achieve the objectives of this course, each student is required to spend a minimum amount of time in each clinical area. Even if all minimum competencies and objectives are demonstrated prior to the end of the course, the student must still complete the minimum number of hours required. All clinical rotations for the semester must be completed prior to the last calendar day of the semester. Each student will spend at least 104 hours in the clinical setting, distributed as follows:

Field/prehospital	48
Emergency Department	40
Anesthesia	16
Total:	**104**

Course Grading: Based on the preceptor evaluation and quality of journaling and patient care documentation, each 12-hour prehospital rotation is worth up to 36 points; each 8-hour ED rotation is worth up to 24 points; and each 8-hour OR/anesthesia rotation is worth 24 points. There are 312 points possible in EMS 250.

Grading Scale:

90–100%	A
80–89%	B
70–79%	C
60–69%	D
59% and lower	F

Submission of Evaluations, Documentation, and Assignments:
Refer to the program *Clinical Handbook and Resource Packet* concerning policies regarding the submission of paperwork.

Course Competencies: Program completion criteria include a minimum number of documented performances of patient contacts in terms of psychomotor skills, patient ages, pathologies, patient complaints, and team-leader skills. Patient contacts may be gained over the three clinical courses in the program, and the opportunity to demonstrate each competency will vary with the clinical assignments for that semester. Satisfactory progress toward the accomplishment of these competencies must be demonstrated each semester. Team-leader skills will be assessed during the third clinical course and during the field internship. Refer to the program *Clinical Handbook and Resource Packet* for a list of required assessment and skill competencies for the EMS program.

Clinical Uniform: Information about the dress requirements for each clinical area can be found in the program *Clinical Handbook and Resource Packet.*

Figure 11-1
Sample Course Schedule

	Date	Day	Time	Topic	Reading	Instructor
1	9/3/03	W	8 A.M.–12 P.M. 1 P.M.–5 P.M.	Introduction and course overview; roles and responsibilities; well-being of the ALS provider; illness and injury prevention; EMS communications; documentation; and medical terminology Homework 1 assigned	*Paramedic Care: Principles and Practice,* vol. 1, pp. 1–107; *Paramedic Care: Principles and Practice,* vol. 2, pp. 250–301	Phillips
2	9/8/03	M	8 A.M.–12 P.M. 1 P.M.–5 P.M.	Ethics, medicolegal aspects of EMS; anatomy and physiology Quiz 1 Homework 1 due	*Paramedic Care: Principles and Practice,* vol. 1, pp. 108–157	Manger
3	9/10/03	W	8 A.M.–12 P.M. 1 P.M.–5 P.M.	Anatomy and physiology Homework 2 assigned	Supplemental reading to be handed out in class.	Johnson
4	9/15/03	M	8 A.M.–12 P.M. 1 P.M.–5 P.M.	Anatomy and physiology; pathophysiology Quiz 2 Homework 2 due	*Paramedic Care: Principles and Practice,* vol. 1, pp. 158–271	Johnson
5	9/17/03	W	8 A.M.–10 A.M. 10 A.M.–12 P.M. 1 P.M.–3 P.M. Lab: 3 P.M.–5 P.M.	Written examination 1 Patient assessment—history-taking and physical examination Lab: Patient assessment Homework 3 assigned	*Paramedic Care: Principles and Practice,* vol. 2, pp. 2–249	Phillips
6	9/22/03	M	8 A.M.–10 A.M. 10 A.M.–3 P.M. Lab: 3 P.M.–5 P.M.	Medication mathematics Pharmacology Lab: Patient assessment Quiz 3 Homework 3 due	*Paramedic Care: Principles and Practice,* vol. 1, pp. 272–365	Manger
7	9/24/03	W	8 A.M.–3 P.M. Lab: 3 P.M.–5 P.M.	Pharmacology Lab: IV access and medication administration Homework 4 assigned	*Prehospital Emergency Pharmacology.* 5th ed.	Manger

#	Date	Day	Time	Topics/Activities	Reading	Instructor
8	9/29/03	M	8 A.M.–3 P.M. Lab: 3 P.M.–5 P.M.	Pharmacology Lab: IV access and medication administration Quiz 4 Homework 4 due	*Prehospital Emergency Pharmacology*, 5th ed.	Manger
9	10/1/03	W	8 A.M.–10 A.M. 10 A.M.–3 P.M. 3 P.M.–5 P.M.	Written examination 2 Airway management and ventilation Lab: Airway management Homework 5 assigned	*Paramedic Care: Principles and Practice*, vol. 1, pp. 500–599	Hartman
10	10/6/03	M	8 A.M.–12 P.M. Lab: 1 P.M.–5 P.M.	Pulmonary disorders Lab: Scenario-based airway management Quiz 5 Homework 5 due	*Paramedic Care: Principles and Practice*, vol. 3, pp. 2–61	Hartman
11	10/8/03	W	8 A.M.–12 P.M. 1 P.M.–3 P.M. 3 P.M.–5 P.M.	Pulmonary disorders Cardiology Lab: "Practice practical"	*Paramedic Care: Principles and Practice*, vol. 3, pp. 62–259	Hartman
12	10/13/03	M	8 A.M.–10 A.M. Lab: 10 A.M.–12 P.M. 1 P.M.–5 P.M.	Written examination 3 Lab: Practical examination Cardiology Homework 6 assigned	Supplemental reading to be handed out in class.	Phillips
13	10/15/03	W	8 A.M.–12 P.M. Lab: 1 P.M.–5 P.M.	Cardiology Lab: Cardiology skills Quiz 6 Homework 6 due	Supplemental reading to be handed out in class.	Phillips
14	10/20/03	M	8 A.M.–12 P.M. Lab: 1 P.M.–5 P.M.	Cardiology Lab: Cardiology skills	Supplemental reading to be handed out in class.	Phillips
15	10/22/03	W	8 A.M.–10 A.M. 10 A.M.–3 P.M. Lab: 3 P.M.–5 P.M.	Written examination 4 Neurology Lab: "Practical practice" Homework 7 assigned	*Paramedic Care: Principles and Practice*, vol. 3, pp. 260–311	Manger
16	10/27/03	M	8 A.M.–12 P.M. 1 P.M.–4 P.M. 4 P.M.–5 P.M.	Lab: Practical examination Endocrinology Allergies and anaphylaxis Quiz 7 Homework 7 due	*Paramedic Care: Principles and Practice*, vol. 3, pp. 312–343 *Paramedic Care: Principles and Practice*, vol. 3, pp. 344–359.	Manger

Figure 11-1
(Continued)

	Date	Day	Time	Topic	Reading	Instructor
17	10/29/03	W	8 A.M.–10 A.M. 10 A.M.–3 P.M. Lab: 3 P.M.–5 P.M.	GI/GU disorders Toxicology Lab: Scenario-based practice	*Paramedic Care: Principles and Practice*, vol. 3, pp. 360–425	Manger
18	11/3/03	M	8 A.M.–9 A.M. 9 A.M.–12 P.M. 1 P.M.–5 P.M.	Written examination 5 Toxicology Environmental emergencies Homework 8 assigned	*Paramedic Care: Principles and Practice*, vol. 3, pp. 426–469 *Paramedic Care: Principles and Practice*, vol. 3, pp. 502–545	Manger
19	11/5/03	W	8 A.M.–11 A.M. 11 A.M.–3 P.M. Lab: 3 P.M.–5 P.M.	Infectious diseases Psychiatric and behavioral disorders Lab: Scenario-based practice Quiz 8 Homework 8 due	*Paramedic Care: Principles and Practice*, vol. 3, pp. 546–605 *Paramedic Care: Principles and Practice*, vol. 3, pp. 606–633	Phillips
20	11/10/03	M	8 A.M.–9 A.M. 9 A.M.–12 P.M. Lab: 1 P.M.–5 P.M.	Written examination 6 Review session Lab: Scenario-based practice and skills review Homework 9 assigned		Phillips
21	11/12/03	W	8 A.M.–10 A.M. 10 A.M.–2 P.M. 2 P.M.–5 P.M.	Trauma systems Mechanism of injury/kinematics of trauma Hemorrhage and shock Quiz 9 Homework 9 due	*Paramedic Care: Principles and Practice*, vol. 4, pp. 2–15 *Paramedic Care: Principles and Practice*, vol. 4, pp. 16–75 *Paramedic Care: Principles and Practice*, vol. 4, pp. 76–121	Hartman
22	11/17/03	M	8 A.M.–10 A.M. 10 A.M.–12 P.M. Lab: 1 P.M.–5 P.M.	Hemorrhage and shock Soft-tissue injuries Lab: Scenario-based practice Homework 10 assigned	*Paramedic Care: Principles and Practice*, vol. 4, pp. 122–169	Hartman
23	11/19/03	W	8 A.M.–11 A.M. 11 A.M.–3 P.M. Lab: 3 P.M.–5 P.M.	Burns Musculoskeletal injuries Lab: Scenario-based practice Quiz 10 Homework 10 due	*Paramedic Care: Principles and Practice*, vol. 4, pp. 170–207 *Paramedic Care: Principles and Practice*, vol. 4, pp. 208–259	Hartman

#	Date	Day	Time	Topic	Reading	Instructor
24	11/24/03	M	8 A.M.–12 P.M. 1 P.M.–5 P.M.	Head and spinal trauma Thoracic trauma Homework 11 assigned	*Paramedic Care: Principles and Practice*, vol. 4, pp. 260–363 *Paramedic Care: Principles and Practice*, vol. 4, pp. 364–411	Hartman
25	11/26/03	W	8 A.M.–10 A.M. 10 A.M.–2 P.M. Lab: 2 P.M.–5 P.M.	Abdominal trauma Special considerations in trauma management Lab: Assessment-based management of trauma Quiz 11 Homework 11 due	*Paramedic Care: Principles and Practice*, vol. 4, pp. 412–443 *PHTLS*, pp. 248–299	Hartman
26	12/1/03	M	8 A.M.–10 A.M. 10 A.M.–12 P.M. Lab: 1 P.M.–5 P.M.	Written examination 7 Pediatrics Lab: Rapid extrication and trauma management Homework 12 assigned	*Paramedic Care: Principles and Practice*, vol. 5, pp. 38–135	Rosen
27	12/3/03	W	8 A.M.–12 P.M. 1 P.M.–3 P.M. 3 P.M.–5 P.M.	Lab: Trauma management skills testing Pediatrics Geriatrics Quiz 12 Homework 12 due	*Paramedic Care: Principles and Practice*, vol. 3, pp. 634–697 *Paramedic Care: Principles and Practice*, vol. 1, pp. 460–477	Rosen
28	12/8/03	M	8 A.M.–11 A.M. 11 A.M.–2 P.M. Lab: 2 P.M.–5 P.M.	Obstetrics and gynecology Communication and documentation Lab: Pediatric management skills Homework 13 assigned	*Paramedic Care: Principles and Practice*, vol. 5, pp. 316–337	Rosen
29	12/10/03	W	8 A.M.–12 P.M. 1 P.M.–3 P.M. 3 P.M.–5 P.M.	Considerations in EMS operations Review session Lab: Skills review Quiz 13 Homework 13 due	Supplemental reading to be handed out in class.	Phillips
30	12/15/03	M	8 A.M.–11 A.M. 12 P.M.–4 P.M.	Final examinations Written and practical (cumulative)		Phillips

Summary

The purpose of this chapter has been to provide you with some ideas and examples of various ways that programs and course offerings can be packaged. Remember, your course or program format may be subject to the guidelines established by state EMS or higher-education regulatory agencies and your institution. As with all the new skills you are acquiring as a beginning instructor, you will probably want to enlist the assistance of, or feedback from, an experienced mentor as you begin to work with program formatting and course scheduling.

REVIEW QUESTIONS

1. What are some advantages and disadvantages of using a semester-based course format?

2. What are the recommended contents of a course syllabus?

3. What are advantages and disadvantages of compressing coursework into a shorter period of time?

12

Program
Evaluation

Learning Objectives

Upon completion of this chapter you should be able to

- State the purposes of program evaluation.

- List the recommended dimensions of program evaluation.

- Differentiate between methods of evaluation and evaluation tools or instruments.

- Distinguish formal from informal evaluation.

- Suggest methods and tools for assessing various dimensions of an educational program.

- Explain the purposes of diagnostic, formative, and summative evaluation.

- Design a program evaluation plan.

CASE
Study

Ty Doyle has just taken a position as the education director with a large, private ambulance service that does its own EMT-Basic courses. The program has been troubled lately, with exam pass rates of 55% to 60% and frequent complaints from the students, their field training officers, and the EMS shift supervisors about the quality of the program. Ty has been unable to find any records to assist him in his analysis of the situation. Ty's supervisor would like to see a report on his desk in 4 weeks detailing Ty's findings and recommendations for improving the program.

Questions

1. What sources of information might be available to Ty to help him make an analysis of the situation?
2. How could Ty collect this information?
3. What can Ty do to get the program back on track?
4. How will Ty know when the program is performing as intended?
5. How can Ty prevent program performance from declining again?

Introduction

In EMS, as in other medical and health sciences programs, there is significant emphasis on educational evaluation, or assessment. Evaluation includes assessment of all aspects of the educational program with respect to the goals of the program. One of the key ways we have of evaluating program effectiveness is to assess student attainment of competencies. We can look at the program's examination scores, standardized examination scores, employment rates, employer satisfaction surveys, and graduate surveys as indicators of educational outcomes. However, we want to find out what educational program components and processes contribute to student achievement, so we are also interested in assessing the quality of teaching, educational materials, clinical sites, laboratory activities, and a variety of other areas. This chapter provides an overview of program evaluation, and Chapter 13 discusses techniques and considerations in student evaluation in particular.

KEY TERMS

bias, p. 185

confounding variable, p. 184

diagnostic evaluation, p. 182

educational assessment, p. 179

educational evaluation, p. 179

evaluation method, p. 184

evaluation tool (instrument), p. 184

formal evaluation, p. 183

formative evaluation, p. 182

informal evaluation, p. 183

Likert scale, p. 185

program evaluation, p. 179

qualitative assessment, p. 186

quantitative assessment, p. 186

summative evaluation, p. 182

Key Areas of Program Evaluation

program evaluation
See educational evaluation.

educational evaluation
See educational assessment.

educational assessment
A process of collecting and analyzing data to determine the status of the educational program with respect to its goals.

Some of the key areas of **program evaluation**—also known as **educational evaluation** or **educational assessment**—include

- Program prerequisites and entry requirements.
- Recruitment and admissions (marketing).
- Faculty instructional effectiveness.
- Student advising.
- Program goals.
- Curricular sequence and structure.
- Course objectives and content.
- Textbooks and learning resources.
- Classroom and lab facilities.
- Instructional materials.
- Cognitive evaluation procedures.
- Psychomotor evaluation procedures.
- Affective evaluation procedures.
- Clinical education.
- Program completion rate.
- Certification/National Registry exam pass rates.
- Graduate competence.
- Graduate employment rate.

A visit to the CoAEMSP website at **www.CoAEMSP.org** will provide information on EMS education program components that are evaluated by the accreditation self-study and site visit. Your state may also have an accreditation process and standards.

PEARLS Some states may have separate accreditation standards from those of the CoAEMSP, particularly at the EMT-Intermediate and EMT-Basic levels.

Program evaluation begins in the program-planning stage.

Preparation for program evaluation begins in the program-planning stage; and evaluation is an ongoing process that takes place throughout the program, not just at its conclusion. It is important that assessment is ongoing so that corrections can be made in a timely manner. Waiting until the next time a program is offered to make needed changes may be disasterous for students of the current program and for the program itself. This is an approach that requires instructional flexibility and open communication with students about the educational process. Planning for evaluation is facilitated by the use of a program evaluation matrix, as shown in Figure 12-1.

Figure 12-1
Program Evaluation Matrix

Dimension of Program Evaluated	Method(s) of Evaluation	Desired Standard	Frequency of Evaluation	Date of Latest Evaluation	Evaluation Results	Standard Achieved?	Action Plan	Person Respon-sible	Date of Follow Up	Results	Reported To
Prerequisites and entry requirements	Faculty and advisory committee surveys	100% agreement of advisory committee	Annually								
Recruitment and admissions	Ratio of applications to student positions	30 students from top 15%	Annually								
Faculty instructional effectiveness	Peer evaluation, student surveys, student outcomes	100% of faculty rated above average	Each semester								
Student advising	Student surveys	100% satisfactory	Annually								
Program goals	Advisory committee survey	100% satisfactory	Annually								
Course objectives and content	Faculty review	100% satisfactory	Annually								
Curricular structure and sequence	Advisory committee, student, and faculty surveys	100% satisfactory	Annually								
Textbooks and learning resources	Faculty review student survey	90% satisfactory	Annually								

Classroom and lab facilities	Faculty review student survey	90% satisfactory	Annually					
Instructional materials	Faculty review student surveys	90% satisfactory	Annually					
Cognitive evaluation procedures	Item analysis, review of face validity	90% satisfactory	Annually					
Psychomotor evaluation procedures	Review of face validity, comparison to NR practical pass rates	90% satisfactory	Annually					
Affective evaluation procedures	Review of face validity	90% satisfactory	Annually					
Clinical education	Student and preceptor surveys, incident documentation	90% satisfactory	Annually					
Program completion rate	No. of students starting/No. of students completing	95%	Annually					
Graduate competence	Employer survey, NR exam pass rate, graduate surveys	100%	Annually					
Graduate employment rate	Graduate survey	100% of those desiring EMS employment	Annually					

Timing of Evaluation

diagnostic evaluation
Assessment of variables of interest prior to an educational intervention for the purpose of directing educational effort.

formative evaluation
Evaluation that takes place while the program is ongoing.

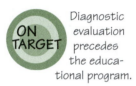

Diagnostic evaluation precedes the educational program.

summative evaluation
Evaluation occurring at the end of a program.

Evaluation should be conducted in three different time frames: prior to program events, during program events, and at the end of a program. Evaluation prior to the start of a program is **diagnostic evaluation.** Pretesting to determine students' retention of BLS knowledge prior to the start of a paramedic program, for example, assists in determining the instructional approach at the beginning of class. Another form of diagnostic evaluation is assessing student academic transcripts to ensure that prerequisites have been met. Diagnostic evaluation prevents having to integrate remedial education components into the course schedule, as would be the case if deficiencies in student BLS knowledge became apparent only several weeks into a paramedic program.

    Formative evaluation takes place during the program. Student surveys, exam and quiz scores, homework grades, preceptor ratings, and practical exams should all be analyzed throughout the program in order to give timely feedback to students on their progress and to make changes in instructional plans before valuable time and resources have been wasted. Formative evaluation is critical to students so that they can assess the impact of their efforts and adjust accordingly. Asking the advisory committee to assess program prerequisites and entry requirements during a quarterly meeting would be formative, as well.

    Summative evaluation takes place at the end of a program with the purpose of comparing actual program outcomes to intended program outcomes. Examples of summative evaluation include the course's final written and practical exams, end-of-course student evaluations of the program, certification exam pass rates, and graduate competence.

Formal and Informal Evaluation

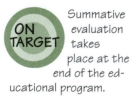

Formative evaluation takes place while the educational program is ongoing.

Summative evaluation takes place at the end of the educational program.

Formal evaluation refers to the planned, often high-stakes, testing and assessments in a program. Formal evaluation includes examinations and end-of-course surveys. Formal evaluation is designed to be measured, analyzed, documented, and, if warranted, acted upon and reevaluated. The use of an outside consultant for program assessment is a type of formal evaluation as well. Peer review of teaching can be either a formal or an informal process, depending upon the program. Peer evaluation is much less threatening if done informally and in a collegial manner.

    Informal evaluation occurs in a variety of ways in an ongoing manner. Noticing puzzled looks on students' faces in response to an explanation of material is a form of informal evaluation, as can be quizzes, homework assignments, and class discussions. Often, students approach the instructor with unsolicited observations, complaints, or suggestions regarding the program. These, too, should be considered sources of information. It is essential that students feel that they can share their observations or concerns with you and perceive that you are willing to listen. Ultimately, the student's observation may or may not be valid, but it is important to keep an open mind and evaluate what the student is saying.

 PEARLS Informal feedback is abundant. Look at students' faces and body language. Follow up on your observations with questions to determine what these clues mean.

formal evaluation
Planned, often high-stakes, testing and assessment. Formal evaluation is designed to be measured, analyzed, documented, and, if warranted, acted upon and reevaluated.

Another form of informal evaluation of learning is the "one-minute paper." At the end of class, ask students to write a brief response to the following questions:

- What was the most useful thing you learned in today's class?
- What was least clear or needs more explanation?

Daily assessment such as this lets the instructor know where to pick up at the beginning of the next class and gives students and instructors alike time to make adjustments before a high-stakes examination. Additionally, it is often easier for students to admit they are still struggling with a concept in this forum than it is for them to verbally acknowledge a general question to the class such as, "Before we move on, is everyone clear on this concept?"

Methods and Tools for Evaluation

informal evaluation
Evaluation that may be unplanned or unsolicited but that provides important information.

We engage in evaluation primarily to allow mandatory reporting to institutional, regulatory, and accreditation bodies, for program improvement, and, often, to justify the training or educational program (Donaldson and Scannell 1986). Knowing this will assist you in identifying meaningful data to collect during evaluation. In general, we want to know three things about our programs:

- What were the participants' reactions?
- What did the participants learn?
- Did the program achieve its goal (better IV start rates, better trauma triage, or whatever the goal of the program was)?

Again, evaluation may be either formal or informal, and this will play a role in your selection of the methods and tools you use for evaluation.

Box 12-1

Examples of Methods and Tools for Evaluation

Program Dimension	Method	Tool (Instrument)
Student learning	Pretest/posttest	Written examinations
On-the-job results	Patient care report analysis	Written report or statistical analysis
On-the-job results	Observation	Written checklist or form
Participant reactions	Survey	Questionnaire

evaluation method
The way in which we collect data, such as observation.

evaluation tool (instrument)
The mechanism for guiding data collection and documentation.

confounding variable
A factor that cannot be ruled out as an alternative or contributing explanation for a finding.

The **evaluation method** is the way in which we find out what we want to know; the **evaluation tool** is what we use to document the data. For example, in assessing student performance on a practical skill, observation by an evaluator is the method; the checklist for that skill is the *tool* that the evaluator uses to record his or her observations. See Box 12-1 for examples of methods and tools used to evaluate particular program elements.

No matter what methods and instruments of evaluation are used, it is often difficult to separate the effects of **confounding variables** from the effects of instruction. (*Author's note:* For example, in 2001, several of my paramedic students in Washington, D.C, were tremendously impacted by the events of September 11. A student on his first field rotation responded to the Pentagon, and others were members of agencies deeply involved with recovery efforts for a period of time afterward. In addition, all students were impacted by the proximity of the event. It is difficult to separate the impact of such an event from the effects of instruction.) An additional example explains why only the first-time attempt at a certification or registration examination is considered a valid indicator of program performance. For students who fail the exam on the first attempt, there is a period in which they are presumably engaging in self-study and/or seeking tutoring and remediation before retesting. In such cases, the effects of initial training are confounded with the effects of additional study. The bottom line is that all evaluations, although useful sources of information, should be seen as part of a bigger picture.

PEARLS Meaningful evaluation requires multiple types and sources of information over time. One piece of data cannot tell the whole story.

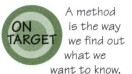

A method is the way we find out what we want to know, such as observation or interview. A tool is what we use to guide and record the findings.

bias
Preconceived notions, which may be conscious or unconscious, that affect the impartiality of a judgment.

Likert scale
A numeric system of rating the relative value of a variable along a continuum of, for example, agree to disagree.

Questionnaires

Using questionnaires to survey students regarding their reactions to an educational program is a common way of collecting data for program evaluation. You are most likely to be able to collect meaningful data if you allow for anonymous response, assess immediately at the end of the program or session, and ask meaningful questions. It is often distressing for new instructors to receive any feedback on their performance that can be perceived as negative. It is important to put this in perspective by remembering that, although student or participant reaction is an important part of evaluation, it is only one perspective. Students can evaluate only on the basis of their prior expectations and experiences and usually cannot accurately assess technical aspects of instruction. For example, although it is common for questionnaires on teaching effectiveness to include items such as, "This program met its stated objectives," studies such as the "Dr. Fox" studies have shown that lecture audiences often perceive that speakers whom they find charismatic or entertaining have met the session objectives, when, in fact, they deliberately did not meet the objectives.

Additionally, there are student factors that can **bias** student ratings of teaching effectiveness, such as a student's level of interest in the subject matter, anticipated grade in the class, personal likes and dislikes, gender, and ethnicity (Koon and Murray 1995). These sources of bias may in turn lead to a "horns" or "halo" effect, in which the rating on one dimension influences the rating on other dimensions. Box 12-2 lists some suggested items appropriate for participant evaluation of an instructional program.

Many questionnaires rely on a rating scale (**Likert scale** or similar scales) based on the degree of agreement or disagreement with statements

Box 12-2

Suggested Items to Assess Student Reaction to Instruction

- To what degree is the content of this session applicable to your job?
- Was the instructor knowledgeable about the subject area?
- Did the instructor present information clearly?
- Were the instructional methods used helpful to you?
- Were the facilities comfortable?
- Was the instructor able to adapt the program to the needs of the participants?
- What part of the program was most helpful to you?
- What part of the program was least helpful to you?
- What changes to the program would you suggest?

quantitative assessment
Measuring variables with respect to a scale of interest.

or scales of excellent, above average, average, below average, poor, etc. Rating scales such as these are considered **quantitative assessments,** because they can be summarized numerically. This often gives an incomplete picture of the program and should be accompanied by some open-ended questions such as, "In your opinion, what was the most helpful part of the presentation?" At the very least, there should be room for general comments. Open-ended questions and records of students' comments are **qualitative assessments** that can give richly descriptive information to illuminate the findings of quantitative analysis.

Possible Explanations for Poor Program Outcomes

qualitative assessment
Collecting and analyzing data that cannot be quantified, such as students' descriptions of their experiences in the program.

Although there is a tendency for program evaluation to focus on the quality of instruction, it is important to remember that there are a variety of factors that can contribute to poor program outcomes. Unless evaluations consider these factors, the reasons for program failure may go undetected. Potential causes of program failure include poor planning, poor timing or scheduling, attractive competitors, inadequate market or marketing strategies, and inadequate programmatic resources or institutional support for the program (Caffarella 1994).

Summary

Program evaluation, or assessment, is critical to continuous improvement of educational programs and may also be mandated by regulatory and accreditation agencies. Program evaluation is multidimensional, including assessment of teaching quality, program planning, program structure, program facilities, and student outcomes. In order for evaluation to be complete and meaningful, there must be a plan for formal evaluation that states the programmatic dimensions of interest, the desired standards, and how and when measurement should occur. Evaluation should also take place informally in an ongoing fashion to ensure that instructional efforts are producing the intended results. Ultimately, the results of evaluation are used to improve the educational program.

REVIEW QUESTIONS

1. List the key areas of program evaluation.

2. When should plans for program evaluation be established?

3. What is the difference between formative and summative evaluation?

4. Give one example each of formal evaluation and informal evaluation.

5. What is diagnostic evaluation?

6. What are the three primary areas of program evaluation?

7. Give an example of something that may be a confounding variable in program evaluation.

Educational
Measurement

Upon completion of this chapter you should be able to

- Differentiate between norm-referenced and criterion-referenced evaluation.

- Distinguish between reliability and validity.

- Discuss the relationship between reliability and validity.

- Define the term *cut score.*

- Discuss considerations in calculating descriptive statistics for exams and assigning grades to student work.

- Compare and contrast quantitative and qualitative methods of student evaluation.

- Explain the importance of constructing a table of specifications for an examination.

- Construct a table of specifications for an examination.

- Provide examples of policies and methods to reduce evaluation-related student aggression.

- Communicate important considerations in test administration.

CASE
Study_____

Shelly Lefevre is sitting in her office with her head in her hands. Her colleague, Dianne Boston, notices and stops to ask Shelly what's wrong. "I just handed back the first exam in my EMT class. The students went ballistic!" "Tell me about it," says Dianne. "Well," Shelly begins. "The students are upset because they feel I asked too many questions on some things, but no questions on other things they thought were important. The average score was 68% and now they want me to grade the exam on a curve. There are two questions that some of the students are sure are asking for the 'wrong' answer, and they're demanding that I give them credit for the answers they gave. What should I do?"

Questions

1. If the students' perception that the test is not representative is correct, how could this have been prevented?
2. Should Shelly grade on a curve?
3. How should Shelly approach the issue of expected answers on the exam that are perceived to be incorrect?

Introduction

Prior to constructing test questions, checklists, quizzes, and other types of evaluation items and instruments, it is necessary that you become familiar with some basic concepts of educational measurement. In this chapter we discuss the purposes of student evaluation, the concepts of validity and reliability in educational measurement, the use of cut scores and grades, the use of quantitative and qualitative methods of measurement, norm-referenced and criterion-referenced procedures, test planning, and considerations in test administration.

KEY TERMS

criterion-referenced measurement, p. 192

cut score, p. 192

formative evaluation, p. 191

index of item difficulty, p. 203

index of item discrimination, p. 203

inter-rater reliability, p. 194

item analysis, p. 202

mean, p. 198

median, p. 198

mode, p. 198

normal distribution, p. 201

norm-referenced measurement, p. 192

qualitative assessment, p. 195

quantitative assessment, p. 195

Reasons for Measuring Student Educational Attainment

**summative evalua-
tion**
Assessment of per-
formance after in-
struction has taken
place.

**formative evalua-
tion**
Assessment of at-
tainment of com-
petencies while the
learning process is
ongoing.

There are a number of reasons why educational measurement, or assessment, is important. First, we want to determine students' performance compared to the predetermined competencies of the program. This
helps us diagnose students' strengths and weaknesses, allows us to assign points and grades, and is one measure of instructional effectiveness.
When we administer a final exam or at least a module exam, we are determining the students' attainment of the terminal performance objectives at the end of a unit of instruction. This is a **summative evaluation.**

Another important use of assessment is to monitor student progress
toward program competencies with quizzes and homework assignments. This measurement of progress is a formative use of evaluation.
Formative evaluation provides feedback to students and teachers alike
so that they can both adapt to increase the effectiveness of the teaching-
learning process in a timely manner. An additional benefit of formative
evaluation is that it can be used to emphasize important ideas, giving
students a sense of the significance of specific concepts in the discipline.
In fact, if a concept is not important, we should not be evaluating student learning with regard to it.

Norm-Referenced versus Criterion-Referenced Measurement

**ON
TARGET**
Evaluation
allows
monitoring
of student
performance
and instructional ef-
fectiveness.

Because EMS is a competency-based field, we must use **criterion-
referenced measurement.** This simply means that we measure students' educational attainment with respect to predetermined levels of
acceptable achievement. The predetermined level of minimum accepted
achievement is referred to as a **cut score,** often expressed as a percentage of points attained on an examination or in a course. These percentages are important because all EMS providers must meet minimum
competency guidelines. In criterion-referenced assessment, every student theoretically can achieve a grade of A, depending upon by how far
they exceed the minimum level of competency. Typically, programs set
their cut scores at around 70% to 75%, and when a letter grade is

necessitated by the institution, the minimum passing grade, or minimum level of acceptable performance, is usually at the C or C− level.

Norm-referenced measurement means that we are interested in how students perform compared to other students rather than how they perform against a standard. When teachers announce that they are grading on a curve, they are engaging in norm-referenced measurement. Norm-referenced measurement necessitates statistical analysis of student scores. The scores are used to calculate a distribution, which can be represented as a curve. Grades are assigned on the basis of the distance of a particular score from the mean (average) score in terms of **standard deviations** (the average distance of scores from the mean). Norm-referenced measurement is great for comparing your height to the height of others in, for example, your ethnic, age, or gender groups. It gives you a sense of how you compare to others. In competency-based fields, however, the use of norm-referenced testing could result in graduating students who cannot perform at entry-level competency simply because they scored better than other students in the class. It could also result in failing students who meet minimum competency levels because they didn't perform as well as their peers.

PEARLS   Because norm-referenced measurement uses overall group performance as the indication of "average" performance, it does not necessarily reflect competence.

Validity and Reliability

Validity refers to the appropriateness of a given means of measurement for determining what it is you want to know. Simply, a valid method or instrument accurately measures what it is intended to measure. For example, if we want to take a patient's blood pressure, we know that the use of a sphygmomanometer and a stethoscope constitutes a valid method of measurement, whereas the use of a pulse oximeter probe is not a valid method of measuring blood pressure. **Reliability** refers to how consistently a method of measurement is correct, or free from errors. For example, if you were to step on a bathroom scale 10 times in 10 minutes and get the same reading every time, the scale would be considered to be reliable. However, if each time you stepped on the scale you got a markedly different reading, the scale would be an unreliable measure of your weight. It is important to note that a measure cannot be valid if it is not reliable. However, a measure may be invalid but quite reliable. For instance, if you were to use the pulse oximeter probe to measure a patient's blood pressure, it would not be a valid measure. But it is quite possible that you might get the same reading consistently, meaning it would be reliable.

standard deviation
The average distance of scores from the mean.

validity
The degree to which a measure actually measures what it purports to measure.

reliability
The degree to which a given measure is dependable, or repeatable, over multiple uses.

Validity

When it comes to written testing, we are most concerned with validity. Gronlund offers the following important points regarding validity:

- Validity is *inferred* from available evidence; it is not measured.
- Validity depends on many *different* types of evidence.
- Validity is expressed by *degree* (high, moderate, or low).
- Validity is *specific* to a particular use of a test or measurement.
- Validity refers to the *inferences drawn,* not the test itself.
- Validity is a *unitary concept.* (1993, 160)

Previously, the testing profession discussed different kinds of validity, such as construct (concept) validity and face (content) validity. Now we consider validity to be a unitary concept. We now refer to different kinds of evidence for validity, such as construct-related evidence or content-related evidence. See Table 13-1 for an overview of the types of validity evidence.

Table 13-1	**Types of Evidence for Exam Validity**	
Type of Validity Evidence	**Description**	**Methods for Achieving/ Assessing Validity**
Content, or "face," evidence	Evidence that an exam adequately represents the content of the domain of assessment.	Examples: Review by a panel of content experts, building the exam from a table of specifications.
Criterion evidence	Evidence that an exam accurately predicts performance related to the actual criterion of interest. For instance, does a test on how to treat poisoning and overdose accurately predict how a student would perform on the actual task?	Determination of the validity coefficient (statistical predictive value) of the test compared to the actual task.
Construct evidence	Evidence that a hypothetical construct exists and that it can be assessed by a particular measure.	A very broad category that considers the arrangement of items on an exam, exam directions, content and criterion evidence, and consideration of a variety of factors besides learning that can affect exam performance.

Establishing validity of large numbers of examination items is a costly and time-consuming endeavor. However, there are things that we, as instructors, can do to increase the chances that a given exam is valid:

- Ensure that the test includes an adequate sample of items to test the objectives of interest.
- Use the proper type and difficulty of items to measure the intended learning outcomes.
- Use properly constructed test items.
- Utilize clearly written items and clearly written exam directions.
- Allow an adequate amount of time for taking the exam.
- Ensure a testing environment free of distractions.
- Keep exam items securely locked away or password protected.
- Do not allow students to take exams with them—once you do, these items are no longer valid in your program.
- Monitor the class closely to discourage cheating.
- Avoid the use of items that are scored subjectively, such as essay items.

Reliability

One particular type of reliability of interest to EMS educators is *inter-rater reliability,* which is typically an issue in laboratory observation, clinical evaluation, and affective evaluation. **Inter-rater reliability** refers to the degree to which different raters using the same instrument agree on the ratings assigned to the same student performance or product. This concept is important in any type of evaluation relying on the observation of student performance and in the evaluation of students' written work, such as journals and essays. Because of the subjective nature of such observations, it is best to use multiple evaluators. The use of behaviorally anchored rating instruments is useful as well. A behaviorally anchored rating scale (BARS) associates a specific description and/or example of the type of behavior with each particular rating on a Likert-type scale.

PEARLS The use of well-constructed behaviorally anchored rating scales for laboratory and clinical evaluation can help increase inter-rater reliability, and thus validity, of measurement.

Figure 13-1
Sample student jour-
naling questions

1. What was the most interesting thing about this clinical rotation?
2. Other than the information already listed on this form, list a mini-mum of two things that you learned from this clinical.
3. How can you apply what you learned today in your practice as a paramedic?
4. Describe the situation today in which you felt the *least* competent.
5. Describe the situation today in which you felt the *most* competent.
6. List at least one goal on which you will focus in order to become entry-level competent as a paramedic. Briefly describe how you will work to achieve this goal.
7. What thoughts and feelings did you experience as a result of this clinical rotation?

Although it is difficult to determine a right or wrong answer, points can be assigned on the basis of the thoughtfulness, insight, and self-evaluation demonstrated by the student. Ideally, students should complete these exercises as self-directed learners, but many students will not go through the exercises unless you grade them on the basis of the thoughtfulness and care taken in answering the questions. In addition to receiving a small percentage of total course points for journaling, students should receive written or, preferably, verbal feedback from you on their writings.

Quantitative and Qualitative Methods of Student Assessment

quantitative as-sessment
Measurement using numeric values.

qualitative assess-ment
Assessment of characteristics of performance that can be described, but not measured quantitatively.

Quantitative assessment refers to any type of student evaluation to which we can assign a numerical score as an indication of student achievement. This is the type of assessment with which instructors are most familiar and the type of assessment most commonly used. Quanti-tative measurement, however, doesn't give the whole picture. **Qualita-tive assessment** is important, but it is often avoided by instructors due to a lack of familiarity and comfort with qualitative methods. Student clinical journals are one type of qualitative assessment (see Fig. 13-1). When asked the right questions to promote reflection, students can pro-vide insightful responses that help tell us about the quality of a particu-lar experience and what it meant to the student. Other qualitative methods include preceptor narratives of student performance and the use of affective evaluation forms. Qualitative assessment is inherently subjective, but its usefulness in drawing inferences can be increased by using multiple raters and carefully designed rating scales.

Planning the Examination: Building a Table of Exam Specifications

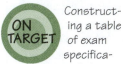

Constructing a table of exam specifications helps ensure that the examination is representative of the learning objectives of interest.

table of exam specifications

A table created to systematically develop an exam representative of the learning objectives.

The primary purpose of building a **table of exam specifications** is to ensure construction of an exam that is representative of the learning objectives for a particular unit of study, thus increasing exam validity. The table of specifications also allows desired distribution of easy, moderate, and difficult exam items. The table of exam specifications is also referred to as a test blueprint or test plan. It is helpful here to work through an example of building a table of exam specifications.

Let's say that we want to construct a test for this text chapter. We begin by looking at the chapter objectives. Of the 10 objectives, we can see that objective 8 is not appropriate to a written test, but it should be tested by assigning students to actually construct a table of specifications. The next step is to decide upon the relative weight of each objective. There is not a particular formula for doing this. Instructors must apply some professional judgment in this step. Although this step is not objective, it does force the instructor to consider all the intended learning outcomes. Validity could be increased at this step by asking the program medical director, program director, or a senior instructor to review the weights you have assigned and discuss his or her thoughts about it with you. The relative weight assigned to each objective is expressed as a percentage. This percentage is then multiplied by the total number of items for the exam. The product is the actual number of items that are written for a particular objective. Once you know how many items you will be writing for each objective, the level at which the objective is written will help you determine the difficulty of each item. Constructing a table of exam specifications can be done efficiently using a Microsoft Excel™ spreadsheet. Table 13-2 is an example of a table of exam specifications for this example.

Students generally ask what is going to be on an exam. It is not a good practice to tell students what is on the examination in more specific terms than that the examination is based on the objectives for the particular unit of study. Nor is it a good practice to tell students during lecture that a given concept will or will not be on the examination. Written testing is a sampling procedure. We make inferences about students' comprehensive knowledge of an area based on a sample of his or her performance. This is much like using a blood sample to infer the characteristics of the total volume of blood in the body. It is not possible to test all the blood in the body, even though we are concerned with the characteristics of the entire volume. Likewise, it is generally not possible to ask every conceivable question that could come from the content. By telling students exactly what is on the exam, you are ensuring that they will study only what they will be tested on and will not focus on learning material that will not (and cannot feasibly be) tested, even though that knowledge is important.

Table 13-2 Sample Table of Exam Specifications for a 25-Item Exam on Chapter 13

	Objective 1	Objective 2	Objective 3	Objective 4	Objective 5	Objective 6	Objective 7	Objective 9	Objective 10	
Relative Weight	0.05	0.15	0.10	0.05	0.15	0.10	0.15	0.10	0.15	Total Weight 1.0
Number of Items	(0.05 × 25) = 1.25 (rounded to 1)	(0.15 × 25) = 3.75 (rounded to 4)	(0.10 × 25) = 2.50 (2 items)	(0.05 × 25) = 1.25 (rounded to 1)	(0.15 × 25) = 3.75 (rounded to 4)	(0.10 × 25) = 2.50 (2 items)	(0.15 × 25) = 3.75 (rounded to 4)	(0.10 × 25) = 2.50 (3 items)	(0.15 × 25) = 3.75 (rounded to 4)	Total No. of items = 25
Number of Items at Level 1 Difficulty	0	1	0	1	0	0	2	1	0	5
Number of Items at Level 2 Difficulty	1	1	2	0	2	2	2	1	3	14
Number of Items at Level 3 Difficulty	0	2	0	0	2	0	0	1	1	6
Total	1	4	2	1	4	2	4	3	4	25

PEARLS Focus students on the learning objectives rather than what will be on the examination. Assure them that the questions asked will be a sample of items based on the objectives they are studying.

Analyzing Exams and Assigning Grades

There are a few simple statistical procedures that you can calculate by hand or using an Excel™ spreadsheet that will give you an overall indication of class performance on the exam and the performance of particular items on the exam in terms of the test's ability to discriminate between higher- and lower-performing students. In this section we consider the descriptive measures *mean, median, mode, range, standard deviation,* and *normal distribution.* We also take a look at the item difficulty and discrimination indices for multiple-choice items. It is important to remember, though, that many of these statistics must be interpreted with caution in a criterion-based situation, because they are norm-referenced measurements.

Exam Descriptive Statistics

There are three common measures of central tendency, or average, used for analyzing class performance on an exam. **Median** is the true middle of the distribution of scores—50% of the scores fall below the median and 50% of the scores fall above the median. The median has the advantage of not being affected by unusually high or low scores. The mathematical average of scores is known as the mean. The **mean** is determined by adding all the students' scores and dividing the sum by the total number of students who took the exam. The mean may not accurately reflect group performance if there are one or two abnormally high or low scores. Because these high or low scores are added in with all the other scores, the mean will be either higher or lower than the median is. The **mode** is the most frequently obtained score. In a normal distribution of scores, that is, the normal *bell curve,* the mean, median, and mode are the same. The **range** of a set of scores is the difference between the highest and lowest scores. See Boxes 13-1 through 13-4 for an illustration of these statistical procedures. Although it is beyond the scope of this text to cover calculating standard deviations, the standard deviation is useful in looking at the spread or variability of scores because it is the average distance of the scores from the mean. In a **normal distribution,** a given percentage of scores will fall within one, two, or three standard deviations of the mean. Knowing the value of the standard deviation allows you to see how

median
A measure of central tendency of scores in which 50% of the scores are higher and 50% are lower than this point. The median is at the middle of the range of scores.

mean
A measure of average performance derived by adding all the students' scores and dividing the sum by the total number of students who took the exam.

mode
The most frequently attained score in a group of scores.

range
The distance between the highest and lowest scores in a distribution of scores.

Box 13-1

Calculating the Mean

Your class of 10 students achieved the following scores on a 100-point exam:

Student 1	92
Student 2	84
Student 3	88
Student 4	62
Student 5	72
Student 6	90
Student 7	88
Student 8	80
Student 9	77
Student 10	75

Total: 808

808/10 scores = 80.8
The mean score is 80.8.

Box 13-2

Calculating the Median

Use the same student scores as in Box 13-1:

Student 1	92
Student 2	84
Student 3	88
Student 4	62
Student 5	72
Student 6	90
Student 7	88
Student 8	80
Student 9	77
Student 10	75

Arrange the 10 scores in order from lowest to highest:

62, 72, 75, 77, 80, 84, 88, 88, 90, 92

When there is an odd number of scores, the median is the score exactly in the middle. For an even number of scores, as here, the two scores in the middle are added together and divided by 2.

In this case, the scores of 80 and 84 are in the middle, with four scores above and four scores below them. The result of adding 80 and 84 and dividing by 2 is 82. The median score is 82.

Box 13-3

Calculating the Mode

The mode of a set of scores is the most frequently obtained score. Arrange the scores as in Box 13-2 from lowest to highest:

62, 72, 75, 77, 80, 84, 88, 88, 90, 92

The score of 88 is the only score that occurs more than once; thus the mode for this set of scores is 88.

Note: If two scores occur with the same frequency, the distribution is called *bimodal*. If more than two scores occur with the same frequency, no mode exists.

Box 13-4

Calculating the Range

Use the same set of scores as in previous examples. The range is the difference between the highest and lowest scores:

62, 72, 75, 77, 80, 84, 88, 88, 90, 92

$$92 - 62 = 30$$

The range of scores is 30.

Box 13-5

The Normal Distribution

The numbers along the y (vertical) axis represent the frequencies with which a score occurs. The numbers along the x (horizontal) axis are standard deviations from the mean. In a normal distribution, 34% of scores are within one standard deviation above the mean, and 34% of scores are within one standard deviation below the mean. This means 68% of scores are within one standard deviation of the mean, 95% of scores fall within two standard deviations of the mean, and 99.7% of all scores fall within three standard deviations of the mean.

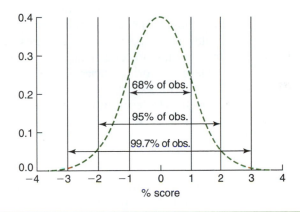

normal distribution
A distribution of scores in which the mean, median, and mode are the same and in which the scores are distributed equally above and below the mean, such that the distribution appears as a bell-shaped curve.

widely dispersed the scores are. Box 13-5 shows a normal curve depicting the standard deviation and the percentages of scores within three standard deviations of the mean.

Grading Scales

In college and university settings you will need to assign grades based on the percentage of points achieved by students. This can be done for each exam or assignment or only at the end of the course. Colleges and universities usually have an established grading scale. One example is as follows:

94–100%   A
90–93%   A-
87–89%   B+

84–86%	B
80–83%	B-
77–79%	C+
74–76%	C
70–73%	C-
65–69%	D
<65%	F

Indices of Item Difficulty and Discrimination

item analysis
The process of calculating for each item on an exam, the difficulty of the item, its ability to discriminate between higher- and lower-achieving students, and the effectiveness of each of the distracters for multiple-choice items.

Item analysis is a process of calculating, for each item on an exam, the difficulty of the item, its ability to discriminate between higher- and lower-achieving students, and the effectiveness of each of the distracters for multiple-choice items. Item analysis is typically used for norm-referenced tests, because in competency-based education our goal is that all learners achieve the competencies. Therefore, there are questions that we must ask that we expect both high- and low-performing students to answer correctly. However, in the microenvironment of your classroom, it can be helpful at times to perform item analysis as a basis of class discussion to improve learning. The steps in performing an item analysis are as follows:

- First, take the third of exam papers with the highest scores and the third of exam papers with the lowest scores. These are the exams you will use in your analysis.
- Using a blank copy of the exam, make a table next to each item as follows:
  - Count the number of students in the upper third who selected each alternative (A, B, C, and D).
  - Count the number of students in the lower third who selected each alternative.

EXAMPLE:

Item 17	A	B	C*	D
Highest third	0	2	6	2
Lowest third	3	2	3	2

*Correct answer

- Determine the percentage of students in the upper and lower thirds who answered the item correctly.

- There are 20 students represented in the table and 9 (6 high-scoring + 3 low-scoring) who answered correctly.
- 9/20 = 0.45 (45%).

index of item difficulty
The percentage of students answering a question correctly.

- The **index of item difficulty** for this group of students is 45%, meaning that 45% of the students answered correctly. The lower the percentage of students answering correctly, the more difficult the item (assuming that the item is valid and well written and the students were given the opportunity to learn the material).

index of item discrimination
A quantitative measure of the ability of a test item to differentiate between high-performing and low-performing students.

- Next, determine the **index of discrimination,** or the discriminating power of the item. This is a measure of the ability of the item to discriminate between higher- and lower-performing students. Remember, in criterion-referenced testing, there are items that we expect all students to answer correctly, so the discriminating power is not always relevant to our purposes.

- Positive discriminating power means that more high-performing students than lower-performing students answered the item correctly.
- Negative discriminating power means that more lower-performing students than higher-performing students answered correctly.
- Items are most effective at discriminating at the level of 1.0.
- A discriminating power of 0.0 means that the item cannot discriminate between high- and low-performing students.

  - Subtract the number of lower-performing students who answered correctly from the number of higher-performing students who answered correctly and divide by the number in each group.
  - In this case

  $$\frac{6-3}{10} = \frac{3}{10}$$
  $$= 0.30$$

  - Thus, in this case, the item has some, but not particularly strong, discriminating power.

- The effectiveness of each *distracter,* an important consideration, can be determined by "eyeballing" the table created for the index of item difficulty.

  - A distracter that attracts more lower-performing than higher-performing students is effective.
  - A distracter that attracts more higher-performing than lower-performing students or one that attracts no one is not effective and should be modified.

Understanding and Managing Student Reactions to and Expectations for Testing

Student Reactions to Poor Test Performance

Evaluations of student performance evoke some predictable emotions and behaviors from students. To a novice instructor, the anger students can express over perceived unfairness in testing can be quite unsettling. Understanding the bases of these reactions and taking a few measures related to exam administration, grading, and return; and grading and return of other performance-assessment measures can help you anticipate and avoid some of these stressful encounters. A poor or lower-than-expected grade on an exam can be a threat to a student's important goals, causing frustration, anxiety, and anger. First, a carefully constructed examination, based on the objectives publicized to the class and principles of good item construction, goes a long way toward eliminating perceptions of unfairness. The following are some other suggestions for reducing strong, negative student reaction:

- Make a policy of requiring that any student complaints about test items be in written format, citing references (such as the course textbook or another credible source) in support of the student's point of view. Be clear with students that you will consider their point of view, but it is not a guarantee of a better grade.
- If you are wrong, admit it and make the necessary corrections.
- Have students discuss the exams in small groups prior to general class discussion. Often, students are less threatened when peers explain their rationale to them.

Student Expectations

Often, students ask questions such as, Can you tell us exactly what is going to be on the exam? Providing this information is not a good practice. An examination can only sample student learning of important material. Testing would be impractical if we were to test every nuance of every objective. The point is, this sample should be an indicator of overall student learning. When students are told "exactly" what to study, that is generally the only thing they study. Thus, students learn only what they can predict they will be tested on. This does not mean that the content of an exam should be a mystery to students. Make clear to students that they will be tested on the objectives covered in a defined period of time.

Summary

The measurement of EMS student competence is a critical aspect of the EMS educator's job. It is important to understand the purposes of student evaluation and the inferences that can be drawn from those evaluations. Because EMS is a competency-based field, the proper means of educational measurement for most purposes is criterion-referenced testing. In criterion-referenced testing, student performance is measured against a prespecified standard, sometimes called a cut score. Norm-referenced testing measures students' performances relative to each other. The methods and instruments we use for educational measurement must be valid and reliable. That is, they must measure what they purport to measure and do so consistently. Creating a table of exam specifications is one means of increasing test validity, because it provides a means of selecting a representative sample of the material to be tested. Finally, the apprentice instructor can be quite dismayed at negative student reactions to poor performance on exams. One of the most important ways of reducing test-related student aggression is to use carefully constructed exams that test the publicized objectives of a unit of learning.

REVIEW QUESTIONS

1. How is norm-referenced evaluation different from criterion-referenced evaluation?

2. Explain the meaning of validity as it relates to assessment.

3. What is a cut score?

4. Describe the purpose of qualitative assessment.

5. Your students have made the following scores on an exam worth 50 points: 45, 47, 35, 39, 37, 50, 42, 41, 45, 49. Calculate the mean, median, mode, and range.

6. Describe weaknesses of norm-referenced evaluation in EMS.

Student Evaluation and Remediation

Learning Objectives

Upon completion of this chapter you should be able to

- Select types of evaluation items appropriate to the measurement of the objectives of interest.

- Discuss the benefits and drawbacks of using particular types of assignments and evaluation items.

- Translate the level and intent of objectives to appropriate evaluation items.

- Write effective selection and supply items.

- Evaluate written examination items against guidelines for effective item writing.

- Differentiate between the method of evaluation and an evaluation instrument.

- Discuss the concept of inter-rater reliability.

- Critique instruments used for clinical, affective, psychomotor, and integration exercise evaluation.

CASE Study____

John Dooley is instructing his first EMT course as a primary instructor. Although he has contributed items for the exams in classes in which he has assisted, he has not written an exam on his own. He has prepared a table of exam specifications to make sure he covers a representative sample of material taught and has decided, based on the objectives, about how many questions for each objective should be at the knowledge, application, and problem-solving levels. Now John must decide what types of items he will construct for the exam. He knows that multiple-choice exams can easily be graded using a computer and that the computer grading system can even calculate the exam statistics and item analysis for him. Yet, he feels that the multiple-choice exam might not tell him everything he wants to know about his students' learning.

Questions

1. Are there types of learning that cannot be assessed with multiple-choice items?
2. What are some of the advantages and disadvantages of using multiple-choice items?
3. What other types of items might John consider using? What are their advantages and disadvantages?

Introduction

Effective educational assessment provides information to the instructor and student. Students are provided feedback on their individual performance, and instructors can note areas of overall weakness in educational attainment as well as identify students in particular need of *remediation*. In order for evaluation of student achievement to be valid and reliable, the methods and instruments selected must be suited to the objectives of interest and the instrument must be well constructed. There are a variety of methods and instruments that can be used, formatively and summatively, to assess student attainment of competency with regard to the stated outcomes of the program. These methods and instruments will vary, depending on whether you are assessing students in the cognitive, affective, or psychomotor domain. In this chapter, you will learn about selecting appropriate methods of evaluation and constructing effective instruments for evaluation. Because the purpose of evaluation is to identify where student achievement lies in relation to program competencies, student remediation is linked to assessment. You will also learn how to assist students in need of remediation and help them develop a plan for remediation.

KEY TERMS

anecdotal notes, p. 229	critical-incident report, p. 230	extended-response essay item, p. 211
bias, p. 232		
checklist, p. 224	evaluation instrument, p. 209	interpretive exercise, p. 211

Written Evaluation of Cognitive Performance

method of evaluation
The procedure used to assess the degree of learning with respect to the variables of interest.

evaluation instrument
The structured document on which observations about student performance are recorded.

selection items
Evaluation items such as multiple-choice and true/false items in which the student must choose one correct answer from a set of choices.

Written evaluation may be formative or summative, consisting of homework assignments, essays, quizzes, and exams. We are mostly concerned here with quiz and test items. For the sake of clarity, it is necessary to distinguish between the **method of evaluation** and the **evaluation instrument.** Cognitive evaluation involves eliciting responses from students with regard to cognitive objectives. We can do this through informal questioning during lectures, assigning homework, or testing. In cognitive evaluation, the written exam is both the method and the instrument. In clinical and lab settings, often the method is observation, but the instrument is a checklist or rating scale.

Types of Written Exam Items

There are two broad categories of test items: selection and supply. **Selection items** include **multiple-choice, true/false, matching,** and **interpretive exercises. Supply items** include **short-answer, restricted-response essay,** and **extended-response essay items.** Each of these types of items has strengths and weakness. In general, selection items are best suited to measure lower-level objectives. They can be used to measure higher-level objectives, but the construction of these items requires considerable time and effort. Selection items allow extensive sampling of multiple objectives and eliminate the bluffing often used in essay items. The scoring is objective and easy, especially if computerized grading is used. When tied to a specific objective (as should be the case), selection items are effective in isolating learning errors. Although selection items are easy to grade, properly constructed items are, contrary to popular belief, difficult to create. In addition, students may guess the correct answer, although this is made less likely by using plausible, attractive distracters.

multiple-choice item
An evaluation item consisting of a stem and approximately four choices, one of which is the correct answer.

true/false item
An evaluation item in which the student must make an evaluation of the correctness of a statement.

ON TARGET Test items must call for the content and level of behavior specified in the instructional objective for the item.

matching item
A type of evaluation item consisting of premises that the student must correctly pair with listed potential responses.

Short-answer items, including fill-in-the-blank-type items, are easier to construct, but again, they are more suited to the measurement of lower-level objectives. Short-answer items have some of the same benefits as selection items, but they have the advantage of eliminating blind guessing of the correct response. On the negative side, students can sometimes bluff their answers on short-answer items, and scoring may be more subjective.

Essay questions are best used to assess student understanding and ability to synthesize information and evaluate situations or propositions. Effective essay items are difficult to construct, can sample only a limited area of knowledge, are prone to bluffing, and grading is difficult and prone to subjectivity.

Matching Test Items to Specific Objectives

If one wants to know if students have accomplished a specific objective, the test item must reflect the behavior called for in the objective, both in content and level. This is critical to the validity of the item. The following examples illustrate this relationship.

EXAMPLE 1

Objective: The student should be able to define medical terminology in his or her own words.

Short-answer item: Define each of the terms listed below in your own words in one or two sentences.

Discussion: Note that the test item mirrors the objective, incorporating all its components. When the item matches the objective, you are then measuring the objective you set out to measure. A multiple-choice item or matching item, for example, would not work well for this objective because the student is selecting from definitions already written and does not have the opportunity to express them in his or her own words.

EXAMPLE 2

Objective: The student should be able to identify procedural steps in patient assessment.

interpretive exercise
A scenario, reading passage, or data display followed by one or more evaluation items that call for the student to analyze, evaluate, and synthesize the information presented.

supply items
Evaluation items in which the student must furnish an answer rather than choosing an answer from an available set of options.

short-answer item
An evaluation item requiring a specific word or phrase to answer a question or complete a statement.

restricted-response essay
An evaluation item calling for an open-ended but more controlled and shorter response than a standard essay question.

extended-response essay item
An evaluation item asking for a relatively open-ended, comprehensive written response.

Multiple-choice item: Which of the following is the first step in patient assessment?

a. Initial assessment
b. Detailed physical exam
c. Scene survey
d. Focused physical exam

Discussion: "Identify" means to recognize something when you see it. This question is suitable for the objective because it is asking the student to identify or recognize the first step when it is situated among other steps, much as you would recognize, or identify, the face of a family member in a crowd.

EXAMPLE 3

Objective: The student should be able to distinguish between patients who meet trauma triage criteria and those who do not.

Selection item: Read each of the following patient descriptions. If the patient meets trauma triage criteria, place an "X" in the blank next to the description. If the patient does not meet trauma triage criteria, place a "0" in the blank next to the description.

Discussion: In this example, the student is being asked to do exactly as the objective indicates. A question asking "Which of the following is a trauma triage criterion," followed by four possible choices, does not test whether the student could differentiate between patients who do and do not meet the criteria—i.e., when the criteria are not explicitly stated.

General Considerations in Writing Test Items

The following are guidelines for avoiding common problems that lower the reliability and validity of test items.

- Avoid unnecessarily difficult vocabulary. Unless the word represents professional terminology, common verbiage decreases the possibility that you are testing the students' vocabulary rather than the objective of interest.
- Avoid complex sentence structure. Often, a couple of shorter sentences provide more clarity than a longer, more complex sentence.
- Avoid ambiguous statements. Have a colleague—or even better, someone not familiar with your program—review your items to help reveal ambiguities. It is often difficult for the item writer to recognize the ambiguity, because he or she is in a particular

mindset when writing the item. The student is not likely to be in the same mindset when reading the item.

- Avoid unclear or poorly reproduced pictures and diagrams (including EKG strips).
- Ensure that the directions for each section of the exam are clear. This is another place in which review by someone else can be valuable.
- Avoid material reflecting race, ethnic, or sex bias. For example, if you are teaching a group of students from the Middle East, a scenario involving an ice hockey injury would handicap the students' understanding of the mechanism of injury. If they are not familiar with the sport, they may be unaware of the presence of sharp blades or the speed at which the puck moves.
- Avoid verbal associations that give away the answer. For instance: The proportion of left ventricular volume ejected during systole is known as

  a. Cardiac output
  b. Ejection fraction
  c. Stroke volume
  d. End-diastolic volume

  Note that the stem contains the clue *ejected,* which is also found only in the correct answer.

- Avoid grammatical clues to the correct answer. For example, make sure the subject and verb agree for all choices, and make sure that you use "a/an" to avoid giving hints about the first letter of the correct answer.
- Avoid using phrases and statements that come directly from the text or handouts, and avoid "stereotyped" phrasing. These give clues to the word for which the examiner is looking, and the student's answer may be more reflective of "seeing the phrase in the mind's eye" than of truly knowing, let alone understanding, the correct answer.
- Vary the length and location of correct answers in multiple-choice items; make sure that all answer blanks are the same size.
- Avoid clues in one item that help answer other items.

Guidelines for Creating Multiple-Choice Items

The general format for multiple-choice items consists of a stem and several alternatives. The stem can either be a question or an open-ended statement, although phrasing the item in the form of a question often makes it clearer. The alternatives include the correct response and incorrect

The statement or question at the beginning of a multiple-choice item is the stem. The incorrect alternatives to the answer are called distracters.

choices called *distracters*. The stem should present a single, clearly formulated problem using simple, clear language. Multiple-choice items read better if as much wording as possible is in the stem and the alternatives are brief. The stem should be stated positively whenever possible, but if negatives are used, they should be emphasized by italic or boldface type.

The intended answer should be clearly the best answer, but the distracters must be attractive and plausible to those who have not learned the material. The use of four choices is recommended. It is difficult to come up with three plausible distracters. When a fourth is added, it is generally clearly not the correct answer and therefore serves no purpose. Using fewer than four choices greatly increases the chances of students guessing the correct answer. Avoid using all of the above and none of the above unless you have an established habit of using these as alternatives that are not always the correct answer. Otherwise, students will recognize that when they see all of the above or none of the above that it is the correct answer.

 PEARLS It is essential that the distracters be both believable and appealing to the uninformed reader.

The following examples illustrate some common problems with multiple-choice items.

EXAMPLE 1 POOR

Do not:

a. Be sedentary if you want to avoid high blood pressure.
b. Drink unfiltered water.
c. Consult a doctor for a cold.
d. Buy drugs from other countries.

Discussion: The stem, Do not, does not give enough information about what is being asked. The distracters are apparently unrelated, and none is clearly correct.

EXAMPLE 2 BETTER

A drug newly approved by the FDA with a classification of 3 means that the drug is a new

a. Molecular drug.
b. Salt of a marketed drug.
c. Formulation or dosage not previously marketed.
d. Combination not previously marketed.

Discussion: The stem in this item provides enough information to answer the question. However, because it is structured as an open-ended statement, the alternatives must be evaluated by reading the stem and completing it with each alternative.

EXAMPLE 3 ALTERNATIVE WORDING

Which of the following best describes an FDA classification of 3 for a newly approved drug?

    a. A new molecular drug.

    b. A new formulation or dosage form not previously marketed.

    c. A generic duplication of a drug already on the market.

    d. A drug that is similar to others already on the market.

EXAMPLE 4 POOR

Which of the following is the longest bone in the body?

    a. Trachea

    b. Colon

    c. Achilles' tendon

    d. Femur

Discussion: The distracters are poor because they are not plausible. Two of them are not part of the skeletal system, and one of them is clearly a tendon, not a bone. The correct answer will be picked not because the student knows it is the longest bone in the body, but because there are no other bones as alternatives.

EXAMPLE 5 BETTER

Which of the following is part of the upper airway?

    a. Pharynx

    b. Trachea

    c. Alveoli

    d. Carina

Discussion: These alternatives call for a higher level of distinction between more similar options. All the choices are part of the airway, and the student must know where the division between the upper and lower airway is and which of the structures is above that level.

Guidelines for Writing True/False Items

True/false items are best for testing knowledge-level cognitive objectives. There is a high probability of guessing correctly, making the diagnosis of learning errors difficult. A more-sophisticated version of true/false items is the corrected true/false item. In this version, if the student selects false, he or she must then correct the statement to make it true or, alternatively, explain why the statement is false. When writing true/false items, include only one concept in each statement. Keep the statement short and use simple vocabulary. Be precise in your statement; it must be unambiguous. Don't use double negatives, and avoid the words that students key in on such as *always, never, sometimes, none, all,* and *only.* The following examples illustrate some common difficulties in the construction of true/false items.

EXAMPLE 1 POOR

True or false:

_____ When you have arthritis you should take aspirin.

_____ Exercise has a positive effect on the body.

_____ No expired medication, even in an emergency, should never be administered to a patient.

_____ Epinephrine, which is favored by experts, is also called adrenalin.

Discussion: There are problems with each of these statements. Should every patient with arthritis take aspirin? Answering true implies that this is the case. Answering false implies that no patient with arthritis should take aspirin. The second statement is relative, as well. What is "positive"? Positive in the short term or the long term? What kind of exercise? The third statement is indecipherable because of the double negative used. The fourth statement contains some truth, but the entire statement is not necessarily true. Epinephrine *is* also called adrenalin, but who are these "experts"? Favored by experts for what use?

EXAMPLE 2 BETTER

True or false:

_____ True/false items are a type of selection item.

_____ Intent must be established to determine whether an action was negligent.

Guidelines for Writing Matching Items

Matching items are usually formatted in two columns. One side lists the premises—the statements that must be responded to—and the other side lists the responses. Use an unequal number of premises and responses to minimize guessing by process of elimination. The responses should be listed numerically or alphabetically to avoid any detectable pattern in the relationship between the premises and responses. When creating matching items, you should include only homogeneous material in each item, much as in writing multiple-choice items. It is essential that the entire matching exercise be on one page of the exam.

EXAMPLE

_____	Alveoli	A. Spasm in asthma
_____	Carina	B. Warms and humidifies air
_____	Epiglottis	C. Protects trachea
_____	Larynx	D. Voice box
_____	Turbinates	E. Sweeps particles up and out of the airway
		F. Site of gas exchange
		G. Point where trachea divides into right and left bronchi

 PEARLS Always use an unequal number of premises and responses for matching items to avoid guessing correctly by process of elimination.

The Interpretive Exercise

The interpretive exercise is frequently used in EMS in the form of written scenarios. The interpretive exercise consists of introductory material, such as a scenario, a text passage, or data display, which the student will have to interpret in order to answer a series of true/false or multiple-choice items based on the material.

EXAMPLE

You have just arrived on the scene of a motorcycle collision in which the motorcycle, carrying two people, entered a curve at high speed and struck a guardrail head-on. Both victims were ejected from the vehicle, over the guardrail. They are about 20 feet down a steep, wooded, overgrown incline. Neither was wearing a helmet. Please answer the following questions regarding this scenario.

1. What additional resources will you need at the scene?

    a. An EMS supervisor
    b. On-site medical direction

    c. Rope-rescue personnel

    d. Triage officer

2. Which of the following actions should you take first?

    a. You and your partner initiate manual cervical spine stabilization for both patients.

    b. Assess the incline to determine if it is safe for you to make patient contact.

    c. Establish medical sector command.

    d. Make sure that both patients have patent airways.

Guidelines for Writing Short-Answer Items

It is often difficult to phrase short-answer items to elicit only one correct response. They should be used only when you want to test at the recall level of performance or when the desired outcome is a computation, such as when you are giving drug dosage and IV infusion-rate problems. Short-answer items present the dilemma of what to do with misspellings and cryptic handwriting. Proper communication in written English is an expectation of professional performance. If you will count off for spelling, make this clear in advance. How much leniency will you allow? For example, is writing *potatoe* instead of *potato* the same as writing *trimmers* instead of *tremors*? Make it clear to students that their handwriting, or preferably printing, must be legible to receive credit for an answer. It is a common ploy for students to write strategic words in an indecipherable manner in order to bluff their way through an answer.

When writing short-answer items, state the item so that only a single, short answer is possible. It is preferable to start with a direct question and switch to an incomplete statement only if greater clarity or conciseness results. When formulating fill-in-the-blank items, leave only one blank and make sure it relates to the main point of the statement. Blanks should be placed at the end of the statement. In addition, avoid clues such as varying blank sizes and the use of *a* or *an*. If you are asking for numerical answers, such as drug dosages, indicate the degree of precision and units to be used in the answer and whether or not work is to be shown. The following examples illustrate the importance of these guidelines.

EXAMPLE 1 POOR

The piece of equipment needed to ensure a good airway is _____.

Discussion: There are several potentially correct answers here: oropharyngeal airway, nasopharyngeal airway, suction, dual-lumen airway device, etc.

EXAMPLE 2 POOR

The _____ of the blood allow the blood to _____.

Discussion: It is unclear what is expected here—there is too much information missing. We could respond with platelets and clot, red blood cells and carry oxygen, etc.

EXAMPLE 3 POOR

_____ is a medicolegal aspect of EMS.

Discussion: Again, there are multiple potential answers here. These could include negligence, confidentiality, consent, abandonment, and many others.

EXAMPLES 4–6 BETTER

The piece of equipment needed to remove blood, vomitus, and secretions from the airway is_____.

The platelets of the blood allow the blood to _____.

The medicolegal aspect of EMS that addresses the EMT who leaves a patient after starting care is _____.

Writing Essay Items

Essay items should be used only to measure complex learning outcomes. The questions should be written clearly and based as directly as possible on the learning outcomes being measured. The question must present a clear task to be performed and provide the guidelines for doing so. It is essential that you specify how many points the item is worth, suggest a length and/or time limit, and provide a framework for answering the question.

EXAMPLE 1 POOR

Discuss the effects of trauma.

Discussion: Numerous lengthy textbooks, review articles, and research studies have been published on this subject. The question is too broad. Should the student be discussing a specific type of trauma? A specific type of patient? The psychological effects? Socioeconomic effects? Physical effects?

EXAMPLE 2 POOR

Why should people stop smoking?

Discussion: The purpose of an essay is to measure the student's ability to synthesize and evaluate complex information. This does not ask the student to elaborate on the negative effects of smoking or the benefits of quitting. If the student answered, "Because smoking is bad for your health," then he or she has answered the question as it is asked.

EXAMPLE 3 BETTER

Compare and contrast hyperglycemia and hypoglycemia in terms of

1. Etiology (2 points)
2. Signs and symptoms (2 points)
3. Speed of onset (1 point)
4. Treatment (5 points)

EXAMPLE 4 BETTER

Criticize and defend the use of PASG in the prehospital setting. Your discussion should include: (1) Relevant studies on PASG, (2) indications and contraindications, (3) complications, and (4) benefits of use. (10 points)

General Guidelines for Assembling a Test

Prior to making copies of the exam, carefully review each item to ensure that it is representative of the table of specifications and that it is appropriate to the outcome being tested. It is helpful to ask yourself what it is you really want the student to be able to do and ask whether the question you have written is really asking the student to do it. Check the difficulty level of the items, based on what action is expected. (See Chapter 10 for a review of verbs representative of each level in the cognitive domain.) Does the difficulty of the item match the difficulty of the objective? Have someone proofread the exam for you to check language and clarity. Your more experienced colleagues can give you valuable feedback on your exams. Although they can be a bit brutal, students will also let you know if exam items are not clear.

PEARLS It is helpful to ask yourself whether the question you have written is calling for the action indicated by the objective.

The test items should be arranged in groups according to type of item and content. For example, part 1 may be multiple choice; in which all cardiac questions are grouped together, all endocrine questions are grouped together, and so on. Within each of these groups, items should be arranged from simple to more complex. Each section or type of question should be accompanied by clear directions:

Part I—Multiple Choice. Read each of the following items carefully. Circle the letter of the best response on your exam sheet and fill in the corresponding bubble on the computer sheet. Clearly mark only one answer for each item.

Instructions such as these will suffice for most purposes, but high-stakes examinations often have more elaborate information, such as the scope and purpose of the test, the number of points possible, the time allowed for taking the test, whether or not students can mark on the exams or use scratch paper or calculators, and whether or not students will be penalized for guessing answers. Make sure that the exam has a place for the student to put his or her name. You may also wish to provide an area in which you can write the score, such as: *Score: _____/60, _____%.*

Other Ways of Evaluating Cognitive Performance

Aside from testing and quizzes, homework assignments can play a role in student learning as well as in evaluation, if properly done. Many of the workbooks and electronic resources available to accompany student texts are aimed at the lower levels of cognitive performance. Other options include having students analyze and present journal articles and assigning defining features matrices, essays, and directed journaling assignments. When asking students to analyze and present journal articles, they must be given specific guidelines and questions to be answered, such as these: What is the importance of the study? What are some limitations of the study? What assumptions did the authors make? How can we use the knowledge generated from this study?

PEARLS Make sure you give students clear guidelines about your expectations for analyzing journal articles. This is often a new type of activity for EMS students.

Box 14-1

Defining Features Matrix

Directions: Compare and contrast placenta previa and abruptio placentae according to the features listed below.

	Placenta Previa	Abruptio Placentae
Definition		
Epidemiology		
Pathophysiology		
Signs		
Symptoms		
Prehospital Management		

A defining features matrix is useful when you want the student to examine two or more ideas or processes that can be confusing, but between which students need to discriminate. The matrix is simply a table that lists the ideas or processes along the top row and the features of interest along the left-hand column. This can be used for examining complaints of abdominal pain, differentiating between causes of altered mental status, etc. Box 14-1 presents an example of a defining features matrix.

Assigned essays involve some of the same considerations discussed for essay questions on exams. You must structure the question, including points you would like the students to address. You must specify the length of the paper. Remember, students can be quite creative, so the length and format should be specified to include the type of font and font size, size of margins, whether single-spaced or double-spaced, and the number of pages. For paramedic students, a 5-page, double-spaced paper with 1-in. margins in 12-point Times New Roman is a significant paper. Also remember to specify whether or not the length includes the references and the editorial style you wish students to use (APA, MLA, Chicago, etc.). You must provide students with information regarding where they can find these styles, as well. Finally, don't assign essays unless you really want to read them to find out what students are learning.

Box 14-2

Directed Journaling Exercise

1. Patient's age, sex, chief complaint:_____

2. Your clinical impression:_____

3. Evidence supporting your clinical impression:_____
_____

4. What labs and diagnostic tests were performed?
   Why?
   How did the results impact further evaluation and treatment?

5. What treatment and interventions were provided to the patient?
   What were the effects of treatment?

6. What was the physician's diagnosis of the patient's condition?
   What is the rationale for the diagnosis?
   What was the patient's disposition?

Directed journaling exercises can be used to promote reflection in both the cognitive and affective domains of learning. The questions used to direct the students' writing should be open-ended and thought provoking. The questions should ask for analysis, synthesis, insight, and, if assessing the affective domain, feelings and responses to situations. Box 14-2 provides an example of a directed journaling assignment.

Creating Performance Assessment Instruments

performance assessment
Assessing student actions, as opposed to written assessment of cognitive achievement.

No matter how well a written exam is constructed, it cannot measure student performance of psychomotor tasks or a student's leadership ability on a call. In EMS we use **performance assessments** to assess both isolated skills and students' abilities to manage complex situations. Performance assessments can focus on the process of the skill or the product of the skill. In EMS, we do both. We are interested in whether the student performs all safety measures needed in a procedure, regardless of whether or not the product is "good." For example, it is critical that the student

Performance evaluation can either consider process or product with respect to student performance.

preparing for synchronized cardioversion take such safety precautions as ensuring the defibrillator is in synchronous mode and that everyone is clear of the patient prior to delivering a shock. Even if there is no harm to the "patient" or classmates, we are concerned if a student does not follow safe procedure. We are also interested in the product of some procedures. For example, after observing students perform all the steps in securing a patient to a long backboard, we will assess the final product by checking that the patient is securely immobilized and in proper position.

Performance assessments are appropriate in the lab and the clinical setting. Each setting has its benefits and drawbacks in terms of assessing student performance. In the lab setting we can control or structure the scenario to include certain features and can standardize the test for all students, but we cannot reproduce the complexities of an actual call. Realistic conditions are difficult to create and require considerable time, labor, and, often, cost. In addition, only one student is assessed at a time, and there tends to be problems with reliability. In creating performance assessments we are concerned with inter-rater reliability—the degree to which two or more observers agree to the ratings of what they have observed. In the clinical setting, we are able to observe the student under real-life conditions, but we cannot ensure that students will encounter particular types of patients or calls. In addition, as with laboratory testing, evaluation can be subjective.

Despite some limitations, performance assessment is a critical component of student evaluation. Regardless of the setting, the method of assessing performance is observation. A variety of instruments may be used to record these observations. Our goal in selecting or designing such instruments is to allow the observer to make particular observations of specific actions.

Considering the Task

Assessment of psychomotor and complex integrated tasks begins with an examination of the task analysis and resulting objectives (see Chapters 9 and 10) as the basis for evaluating performance. It is essential that the conditions of the performance evaluation elicit the actual behavior called for by terminal performance objectives. For example, students often try to "talk" their way through procedures, saying what they would do, but they hesitate to actually perform the skill step of, say, checking the pedal pulse. If the desired action is for the student to *perform,* then the assessment conditions must require him or her to perform, not talk about the skill. Otherwise, we might find that the student knows he or she should check the pedal pulse, but we have no idea if the student even knows he or she has to take off the patient's shoe to check it.

Students often try to talk their way through procedures. Procedures can only be learned by the student and evaluated by the instructor if the student is required to actually perform what is expected.

Checklists

checklist

An instrument used to guide evaluation of a task.

When teaching skills, the details of the task analysis are important. In assessing skills, listing too many items on a **checklist** becomes cumbersome. The evaluator may become so focused on reading the checklist that he or she misses steps performed by the student. A skill or performance checklist should include the main steps of the task and any critical steps and criteria. For example, Gronlund (1993, 123) suggests that the following criteria be considered in evaluating task performance:

- Rate or time—such as ventilating a patient at a rate of 12 breaths per minute or beginning transportation of a trauma patient in under 10 minutes in a scenario.
- Error—such as preparing a patient care report with three or fewer errors.
- Precision—such as calculating a drug dosage to $\frac{1}{100}$ of a unit of measure.
- Quantity (or frequency)—for example, rechecking patient vital signs every 5 minutes.
- Quality—for example, neatly bandages a soft tissue injury, or performs lifts using correct body mechanics.
- Sequence or order—the checklist should specify whether or not the sequence of steps is critical.
- What material (or equipment) should be used—such as specifying the use of a particular type of short spinal-immobilization device.
- Safety—the checklist should include required safety measures as well as the actual steps of the task or procedure.

The skills checklists for BLS- and ALS-level skills required by the National Registry of EMTs can be found on the organization's website at **www.nremt.org** and can also be found in many textbooks. However, there are other skills and complex performances on which you may want to evaluate your students that are not included in the National Registry skill sheets. Box 14-3 provides an example of a skill checklist.

Box14-3

Skill Checklist

Arterial Blood Gas Sampling—Radial Artery

Directions to the evaluator: Place a checkmark in the appropriate column to indicate whether the student performed the step; performed it incorrectly, incompletely, or in incorrect sequence; or did not perform the step at all. Please provide comments about your ratings.

Step	Performed Correctly (1 point)	Performed Incorrectly, Incompletely, or in Incorrect Sequence (0 points)	Not Performed (0 points)	Comments
*Prepare equipment.				
*Explain procedure to patient.				
*Check for contraindications.				
*Perform Allen's test.				
*Position extremity.				
*Take appropriate BSI.				
*Cleanse site with antiseptic solution.				
Palpate radial pulse just proximal to puncture site.				
Slowly advance the needle through the skin at a 45° to 90° angle until blood appears in the collection syringe.				
Obtain a 1- to 2-mL sample.				

Troubleshoot arterial puncture if appropriate.				
Withdraw the syringe and immediately apply firm pressure to the puncture site with a gauze pad for 5 min.				
Ask examiner to act as assistant in maintaining arterial pressure; then expel air from syringe.				
Stopper syringe.				
Gently rotate syringe to ensure heparinization of sample.				
Label sample with patient's name, date, time, patient's temperature, and amount of oxygen being administered.				
Bandage site.				
Explain method and frequency of reassessment of the puncture site.				

*The sequence is not critical as long as all steps with an asterisk are completed prior to arterial puncture.

Rating Scales

rating scale
An instrument used to assign a value to student performance.

Although checklists allow the observer to record whether or not a skill step was performed, a rating scale allows recording how well something was performed. **Rating scales** are often used to evaluate student clinical performance. Such ratings are subjective, but inter-rater reliability can be increased by using behavioral anchors with the ratings. This gives the evaluator an idea of what should be included in, say, "professional appearance" ratings of 1, 2, 3, and 4. As indicated by the use of professional appearance here, rating scales can also be used for affective evaluations. Box 14-4 provides an example of a rating scale.

Box 14-4

Behaviorally Anchored Rating Scale

PRECEPTOR EVALUATION OF STUDENT PERFORMANCE

Directions to the Preceptor:

Please use the rating scales below to describe your evaluation of the paramedic student to-day. Please discuss the rationale for your evaluation with the student and help the student identify strengths and areas for further development. There is space provided for additional comments and signatures. When you have completed the form, place it in the envelope provided, seal the envelope, and sign your name across the seal. Return the envelope to the student.

Part A: Affective Domain

1. Preparedness: The student arrived on time with ink pen, stethoscope, eye protection, penlight, and required paper work and identification.

0	1	2	3	4
More than 15 min late and/or no equipment	10–15 min late and/or missing 2–3 items above	5–10 min late and/or missing 1–2 items above	Arrives at the last minute; missing 0–1 item above	On time, not rushed, has all equipment

2. Professional appearance: The student is dressed in proper uniform and is neat in appearance.

0	1	2	3	4
Not in uniform, poor hygiene	Uniform is dirty, wrinkled or has holes in it. Poor judgment in jewelry and/or makeup	Uniform acceptable, could improve by polishing boots, etc.		Uniform clean and neat. Student well groomed

3. Initiative: The student demonstrates interest in EMS through actions and interactions with evaluator.

0	1	2	3	4
No questions asked, minimal participation when requested	Asks few questions, minimal participation and initiative.	Asks questions or studies, good participation if asked but little initiative	Asks questions, studies in down time, active participation.	Asks questions, curious, takes initiative, and follows through.

4. Conduct: The student interacts with patients, families, and coworkers in a respectful and empathetic manner and demonstrates respectability and professional ethics.

0	1	2	3	4
Violates the rights of others; cannot be trusted with the property of others. Violates privacy and confidentiality. Is rude or disrespectful.	Shows little interest or ability in interacting with patients or coworkers.	Interacts with patients and coworkers but lacks in empathy and/or professionalism.	Overall conduct adequate. Needs self-confidence and assertiveness.	Initiates therapeutic communications with others. Puts patients' needs above own self-interest. Demonstrates an attitude of professional collegiality.

5. Careful delivery of service: The student follows policies, procedures, and protocols, and uses appropriate safeguards in the performance of duties.

0	1	2	3	4
No regard for the safety of self, patients, or staff. Disregard for policies, procedures, protocols.	Minimal regard for safety, policies, and procedures	Inconsistent in use of safeguards.	Needs minimal supervision to perform safely and adhere to policies and procedures.	Exercises due caution in the performance of duties and follows policies, procedures, and protocols.

Part B: Psychomotor Domain
1. The student demonstrates proficiency in skills performed.

0	1	2	3	4
Does not know what skill is indicated and if prompted cannot perform it.	May know what skill is indicated but cannot perform it.	Knows what skill is indicated but performs poorly without instruction.	Knows skill is indicated, performs correctly but needs to increase speed.	Knows skill is indicated. Organizes the task efficiently, performs accurately and without hesitation.

Part C: Cognitive Domain
1. Knowledge: The student can recall common terms, facts, principles, and basic concepts in EMS.

0	1	2	3	4
Significant deficits in knowledge; e.g., cannot use basic medical terminology.	Somewhat limited recall of facts and principles.		Good recall of most facts and concepts, given the current point in the course.	Outstanding recall of principles and theories.

2. Problem solving: The student uses knowledge to solve a previously unencountered situation.

0	1	2	3	4
Unable to recognize problems.	Recognizes the problem but cannot solve it.		Identifies the problem and takes some steps toward solving it but needs guidance.	Identifies problems and can independently devise a plan to solve the problem.

3. Evaluation: The student can judge the appropriateness of actions and can defend his/her decisions.

0	1	2	3	4
Cannot give a rationale or explanation for actions or decisions.		Attempts to defend his or her decisions or actions but does not provide a defensible argument.		Provides a sound rationale for decisions and actions.

Please use the space below to write any additional comments and suggestions for further development of the student's potential.

Preceptor Signature_____ **Title**_____ **Date**_____
Student Signature_____ **Date**_____

Anecdotal Notes or Critical-Incident Reports

Observations may also be recorded in written form, detailing student performance. **Anecdotal notes** are useful as a supplement to checklists and rating scales. **Critical-incident reports** are appropriate when an unusual event (positive or negative) occurs that cannot be explained by standard forms. These instruments are subjective and rely upon that to which the evaluator pays attention without the guidance of a checklist or rating scale. Box 14-5 provides an example of anecdotal notes, and Box 14-6 shows a critical-incident report.

Box 14-5

Anecdotal Notes

On September 19, 2004, paramedic student Michael Simmons arrived at 0640 hours for his 0700 field clinical rotation at Station 4. His professional appearance was impeccable and he demonstrated exceptional initiative in participating in house duties. At 0900 Mr. Simmons witnessed one of the engine crew go into cardiac arrest while running on the treadmill in the station. Mr. Simmons acted immediately, calling for help and bringing the defibrillator and resuscitation bag from the ambulance. The patient was in ventricular fibrillation, and Mr. Simmons successfully defibrillated him on the first attempt. Mr. Simmons continued to act as team leader throughout resuscitation and transport of the patient. Mr. Simmons demonstrated extraordinary professionalism and presence of mind in taking control of this situation.

Respectfully submitted,

Private G. Longerich, Dranesville Fire Department, Medic 4 A-shift

cc: D. Arnold, A-shift EMS Captain, Dranesville Fire Department

D. North, clinical coordinator, Forest Grove Community College EMS program File

---

critical-incident report
A written document addressing a significant unusual occurrence during the educational program.

Portfolios

A **portfolio** is a collection of student work samples. This is a method by which the student can demonstrate accomplishment as well as being an instrument of evaluation. This is particularly useful in collecting student clinical documents, such as directed journaling assignments, preceptor evaluations, and student patient care reports or case studies. This gives the instructor a mechanism for reviewing the student's clinical progress and allows the student to see how he or she is progressing over time.

Assessing the Affective Domain

Assessing the affective domain is relatively new in EMS. It is also the most difficult of the three areas of student evaluation. Although we are interested in the student's values, we must rely on observed behavior,

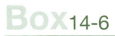

Critical-Incident Report

Critical-Incident Report

Preceptor Name_____   Date_____

Preceptor Telephone_____ Time of Incident_____

Clinical Site and Unit_____   Student _____
Others involved or
present_____
_____

Description of Event

[blank lined box]

Preceptor Signature_____
_____

To be completed by EMS Program Faculty

Date Received by Clinical Coordinator_____

Date Reviewed by Program_____ Reviewed by:_____

Actions or Recommendations_____
_____

portfolio
A collection of significant student work.

Anecdotal notes and critical-incident reports are used to document occurrences that are significantly unusual and cannot be documented on standardized forms.

bias
Prejudice.

social perception
The process by which we attempt to make sense of others and what they do.

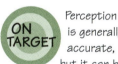

Perception is generally accurate, but it can be prone to specific types of errors.

from which we must draw conclusions about the student's values and attitudes. Here, more than in assessment of cognitive and psychomotor learning, *bias* and *perception* can greatly impact ratings of student behavior. It is worth examining some of the more common forms of **bias** in the process of social perception.

Social perception is the process by which we interpret others' behaviors. Social perception is an ongoing process of which we are seldom aware. Although perception is fairly accurate, it is prone to errors, as well. Some of the common perceptual errors include fundamental attribution error, the horns (or halo) effect, the similar-to-me effect, and stereotyping.

Fundamental attribution error is the tendency for people to attribute the cause of another's behavior to intrapersonal characteristics rather than to situational influences. That is, if a person behaves in a particular way, we are more likely to assume the behavior is a result of personality or disposition rather than something going on outside the person. This effect is heightened when we see the person act in the same way across different situations and when other people do not act the same way in the same situation. For example, if one of your students complains bitterly about the coffee from the vending machine but other students don't, we are more likely to attribute the complaint to the student's being difficult to please. Perhaps, though, other students do not like the coffee, either, but choose not to complain about it for various reasons, such as it meeting their expectations for vending machine coffee.

The halo (or horns) effect occurs when a positive (or negative) impression of one attribute of a person colors our perception of his other attributes. For example, Alexander, Limmer, and Monosky (2002) found that attendees at a preceptor workshop rated the overall videotaped performance of patient assessment lower when the actor portraying an EMS provider was dressed sloppily than when he was dressed neatly, though the patient care performance was the same.

The similar-to-me effect occurs when evaluators rate more highly those students whom they see as being more similar to themselves in important ways. The evaluator is better able to empathize with the student's (or employee's) general behavior and beliefs. Because of this, the evaluator is more likely to rate specific behaviors more positively.

Finally, stereotypes can also lead to errors in perception and thus errors in ratings of student behavior. Stereotypes are a type of schema that serve a useful purpose unless our stereotype consists of overgeneralizations that lead to inaccurate judgments about people. It is important that we evaluate students' behavior on its own merits and not on the basis of whether the student is one gender or the other, because they belong to a particular ethnic or racial group, or even because they belong to a particular occupational group.

Baron and Greenberg (2000, 64–65) offer the following recommendations for reducing bias in our judgments of others.

- Don't overlook external causes of others' behavior or performance.
- Identify your own stereotypes. When evaluating a member of a group about which you hold the stereotype, ask yourself whether you are evaluating the person as an individual or as a member of a group.
- Use objective information, such as what the person did, rather than making implications about, for example, what the person intended or thought, to make your judgments.
- Avoid jumping to conclusions. Keep an open mind about subsequent behavior.

The 1998 Paramedic National Standard Curriculum (NHTSA) contains affective evaluation instruments and examples of affective evaluations. You can find these at **http://www.nhtsa.dot.gov/people/injury/ems/nsc.htm** .

Evaluating affective behavior is a sensitive area, should the need to counsel a student about his or her behavior arise. Remember, the purpose of assessing affective behavior is to monitor progress toward the attainment of professional characteristics. In general, the qualities of concern—for example, punctuality—should have been noted by more than one observer and under various circumstances. When counseling the student, more than one faculty member should be present, and the observations should be delivered tactfully and in a nonaccusatory manner. This is an opportunity to help the student see how he or she is perceived by others and what his or her behavior tells others. Obviously, some behaviors, such as plagiarism, theft, sexual harassment, or ethics violations, are disciplinary in nature and are handled in another forum. That aside, students may truly be astounded that their behavior was perceived as it was and appreciate the insight; others, no matter how tactfully you deliver the information, will be defensive and angry. No matter how angry and argumentative a student becomes, it is essential that you stay calm. Chapter 18 further addresses handling various student issues.

PEARLS The nature of affective evaluation requires that you meet in person with students to discuss their progress.

Remediation

Remediation is a process of assisting students who have not met the expected competencies of the educational program in identifying and correcting deficiencies. Simply, a deficiency occurs when actual performance

remediation
Identifying and assisting students in learning material that was not initially learned through the curriculum.

is beneath the level of acceptable performance. Occasionally, an examination, either written or practical, will reveal that the majority of students did not perform well with respect to specific objectives or even in specific content areas. With such a systematic deficiency in performance, there is likely to be a problem with instruction or with the evaluation instrument. In this instance, it is important to examine the teaching methods and content delivered in that area. As the course instructor, you must build time into the class schedule to correct the deficiencies. In other instances, one or a few students are struggling, whereas the majority of the class is performing as expected. In cases such as this, you should meet with the student individually to discuss potential causes of the deficiency.

Many of the issues surrounding student performance should be addressed in your program policies. The prerequisites for admission to the program, the performance standards, and the consequences of failing to meet them should be clearly stated. Any policies addressing retests should also be stated. Along with this, it is important to realize that, as an instructor, you do owe your students a certain amount of availability outside of class time to discuss class issues. At times the student may take the initiative to come and talk to you prior to your having enough evidence to detect a problem. At other times, you will need to ask the student to make an appointment to come and talk with you about his performance. Beyond recognizing straightforward educational problems and solutions for remediation, an introductory instructor course cannot prepare you to diagnose the student's difficulty or to create a complex plan of educational counseling in learning strategies. One of the benefits of being part of a program conducted within an academic institution is the availability of student services to assist the student in discovering his or her learning style and effective study strategies. Finally, should the student attribute his or her performance to a learning disability, the student should be referred to the appropriate services for testing and provision of accommodations (see Chapter 3).

ON TARGET

A learning contract is an agreement between the student and the instructor that specifies what the student has committed to in terms of educational effort as well as the expectations for academic performance and consequences of not meeting those expectations in a given time period.

It is important to discuss with the student his or her perceptions of the problem and the factors that may be contributing to it. For example, has there been a recent change in the student's situation that has caused previously good performance to suffer? Or is this an ongoing performance deficit? Has the student performed well in other situations? Does the student feel that he or she is being evaluated unfairly? Perhaps you and the student together can identify some of the difficulties. It is possible that the student will relate to you that he or she has never had good study habits and needs help in this area. Perhaps the student will admit that he or she hasn't put forth the effort needed. But you should also be prepared for the occasional student who directs anger at you because you are perceived to be the barrier to the goal of successfully finishing the course.

Some of the suggestions that might be appropriate in given situations include suggesting that the student find a study partner or join a study group. You can suggest supplementary texts that the student might find more appealing and can keep a list of former students who are interested in tutoring. Remember, your role is to facilitate the student's learning, but the student must take ultimate responsibility for his or her own learning. In any case, it can be helpful with some students to enter into a learning contract. This can be a simple written agreement between you and the student specifying to what the student has committed in terms of educational effort. This could include the student's agreeing to spend 3 hours a week with a tutor, completing enrichment exercises, or committing to meeting with a study group twice a week. The agreement should also make clear the expectations for academic performance and the consequences of not meeting those expectations.

Summary

Educational assessment is an important process designed to assess student achievement relative to the stated competencies of the educational program. Formative evaluation provides both students and instructors with feedback so that any needed changes in teaching methods or study habits can be made in a timely manner. Summative evaluation is a measure of the overall effect of instructional efforts in preparing students for entry-level competency at their level of practice. The methods and instruments used for evaluation must be suited to the objectives of interest, and the instrument must be well constructed. Methods and instruments will vary, depending on whether you are assessing students in the cognitive, affective, or psychomotor domain. Educational evaluation is also a key step in creating student remediation plans.

REVIEW QUESTIONS

1. For what purposes are essay items best used?

2. What is the difference between a method of evaluation and an instrument of evaluation?

3. How can the possibility of students getting a true/false item correct by guessing be reduced?

4. How can the horns/halo bias affect evaluation of student performance?

5. What is fundamental attribution error?

6. What actions should be taken if your class, as a whole, does not perform particularly well on an examination?

Selection of Materials and Media

Learning Objectives

Upon completion of this chapter you should be able to

- Apply criteria for distinguishing between high- and low-quality teaching and learning resources.

- Discuss considerations in the selection of teaching materials and media and student reading material.

- Describe the uses, benefits, and potential drawbacks to the use of audiovisual materials in teaching.

- Employ principles of effective use of educational materials and media.

- Compare and contrast the advantages and disadvantages of different formats for audiovisual presentations.

CASE Study____

Micki Fischman is the program director of the EMS program at Calverton Community College. Her instructors have provided her with their requests for training equipment for the next fiscal year. Micki must make decisions about which of the requests can and should be honored and create a budget for these items.

Questions

1. What questions must be answered before Micki can decide which equipment should be purchased for the coming fiscal year?
2. What sources of information will Micki need to determine the costs of the equipment to be purchased?

Introduction

The variety of instructional resources, materials, and media available for teaching in EMS has increased dramatically in the past several years. Resources and materials can be as simple as a handout or as sophisticated as programmable interactive mannequins and simulators. There seems always to be a temptation to select the newest, most high-tech, most expensive equipment, but it is important to understand that the most complicated, newest, most expensive, or otherwise seductive materials are not always the most functional or best suited to your instructional purposes. It is important that you know the advantages and disadvantages of a variety of materials and media, the purposes for which they are suited, their limitations, and criteria for making decisions about investing in them. In this chapter you will learn about selecting textbooks, training equipment, and audiovisual materials as well as some principles for creating your own materials.

KEY TERMS

Flesch-Kinkaid Grade Level Score, p. 240

Gunning's Fog Index, p. 240

pedagogical features, p. 241

reading level, p. 240

Textbooks

One of the first things to learn about textbooks is that a textbook is not a curriculum or a course. Textbooks are adjuncts to the curriculum used for the purposes of providing students with information prior to class to serve as a framework for in-class activities, a reference for information outside of class, and a source of information to supplement or review in-class information. There are a variety of EMS textbooks available from several publishers for each of the nationally recognized levels of EMS practice as well as for specialty topics such as pharmacology, EKGs, anatomy and physiology, pathophysiology, rescue, incident command,

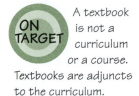

response to terrorism, and other areas. It is critical that you review any text you are considering requiring for your students. The same publisher may offer several choices of textbooks for a particular level of training or topic. Each of these generally has a different approach and may be different in reading level, depth and breadth of information, pedagogical features, and student and instructor resources and supplements. You can contact the publisher representative for a particular textbook to request an instructor desk copy if you are considering the use of the textbook. If you don't know who the representative is in your area, you can either find or inquire about who it is on the publisher's website.

Guidelines for Selection of Printed Materials

Content

Most EMS textbooks are based directly on the NSC as a minimum, and many use the lessons and objectives of the NSC as the structural foundation of the text. Yet, different areas or different objectives within an area may receive more or less emphasis. It is important to consider the depth and breadth of coverage of cognitive, affective, and psychomotor content. The content must be current, relevant, and accurate. Enrichment material beyond the core content should be identified as such. The level of difficulty of the material must be consistent with the goals of the program. For example, an ALS textbook with very in-depth pathophysiology may be appropriate for paramedic students but not for intermediate students.

Style

The writing style should engage the reader and avoid bias toward or against a particular group (e.g., fire-based versus hospital-based EMS, male providers versus female providers, stereotyping patients in scenarios, etc.). Ideas must be clearly organized and identified and flow logically. The language should be clear, accurate, and precise. Unnecessary wordiness obscures the meaning of the message. Texts that connect with students' experiences are more likely to engage students. It is helpful if students can identify with scenarios and the characters in them.

Physical Characteristics of the Book

Students prefer books that are smaller in size, lighter, and more compact. This improves the portability of the text so the student can make maximum use of his or her time. Pages printed on matte paper, rather than glossy paper, are easier on the eyes. Minimum font size should be 12-point Times New Roman, but larger print may be desired to prevent eyestrain.

Reading Level

reading level
An indication of the reading skills needed to read and comprehend text passages and articles.

One of the keys to selecting a textbook for your course is to know your audience. Are you teaching a first-aid or first-responder course to high school students, a community group, or work group? Or are you teaching an EMT-B or paramedic course in a community college or university? The **reading level**—i.e., the reading skills needed to read and comprehend—of these groups can vary. The average American reads at about the sixth- to eighth-grade level. Attempting to use a textbook at too high a reading level can frustrate the learner and interfere with the learning process. The publisher may be able to provide you with information about reading level, or there are a variety of quick assessments of reading level you can apply, many of which can easily be found online (Gunning's Fog Index, Flesch-Kinkaid Grade Level Score, etc). Medical terminology generally raises the reading level of textbooks and may or may not be included in various assessments of reading level. It is also important to consider reading level when assigning outside readings such as journal articles and when writing exams. In terms of materials you develop yourself, Microsoft Word® provides an option to use the Flesch-Kincaid Grade Level Score and the Flesch Reading Ease Score to determine the difficulty of the text. First, you must enable the option by clicking on Tools, Options, Spelling and Grammar, and then clicking on the option to display readability statistics. Select the passage you want to analyze and perform a spelling and grammar check. When Microsoft Word finishes checking spelling and grammar, it displays information about the reading level of the document.

Flesch-Kinkaid Grade Level Score
A procedure used to calculate a grade-based indication of reading difficulty.

Gunning's Fog Index
A simple method for quickly determining the readability of text passages and articles.

The **Flesch-Kinkaid Grade Level Score** goes from 1 to 12 to reflect the grade level at which the reader has to read in order to read the passage effectively. Again, the average adult in the United States reads at about the 8th-grade level. The Flesch Reading Ease Score is a number from 1 to 100. The higher the score, the easier the reading passage is. To meet the abilities of the average person, the Reading Ease Score should be between 60 and 70. **Gunning's Fog Index** is simpler to calculate. Select several paragraphs from a document or text. Count the number of sentences in the paragraph. Count the number of words with three or more syllables, but exclude words in which *es* or *ed* form the third syllable. Also exclude hyphenated words and compound words such as newspaper. The average sentence length is the total number of words in the paragraph divided by the number of sentences in the paragraph. For example, if a text passage or paragraph has a total of 100 words and there are 5 sentences in the passage, the average sentence length is 20 words. The percentage of "big words" is calculated by dividing the number of words with three or more syllables by the total number of words in the passage. Assuming that there were 15 big words in the passage, the percentage of big words would be 15/100, or 15%. Finally, add the average sentence length to the percentage of big words and multiply by 0.4. The result is the Fog Index score. In this case, $(20 + 15) \, 0.4 = 14$. The score reflects the expected reading ability of a person with that number of years of schooling. Fourteen means the reading level is that of a person who has graduated from high school and has 2 years of college education. Add together the scores for all passages evaluated and divide by the number of passages selected to obtain the average readability of the material. See Figure 15-1 for an example.

Decisions on texts should not be based solely on reading level. Indices of reading difficulty cannot tell you how complex the ideas conveyed through language are. The reading indices are based on the numbers of words in a sentence and the numbers of syllables per word. Therefore, sentences and words may be simple, yet the concepts may be quite complex. The use of medical and scientific terminology raises the reading level, but because it is unavoidable, it is the underlying level of readability with which we are concerned. Try to select passages without medical or scientific terminology. Neither can the indices tell you if the vocabulary is appropriate, whether the writing style is engaging, or even if the material is presented in a logical sequence.

Pedagogical Features and Technical Design

pedagogical features
Textbook features that assist students in summarizing, analyzing, and applying text material.

Pedagogical features of textbooks refer to the illustrations, tables, diagrams, charts, review questions, and other items that help summarize information and stimulate the reader to process the information. These features are not only appealing to visual learners, but are helpful to all learners. Technical design refers to the structure and organization of the text.

The content should be introduced in a table of contents. The structure of the content should be clarified through the use of chapter titles (instead of just numbers), headings, subheadings, introductions, and summaries or conclusions. Each chapter should state the objectives to be learned and provide an overview of the content. Key words should be introduced in bold type. There should be sufficient room in the margins, or "white space," to improve readability. Finally, the content must be arranged in "chunks" of suitable size so that the student can reflect upon material incrementally.

Illustrations and photographs should have a meaningful purpose as an adjunct to the text. That is, they should focus the student on the concepts rather than providing diversion from it. They should be clear and of high quality and should be annotated or clearly referred to in the text.

Figure 15-1
The Gunning Fog Index
in Use

Paragraph 1

Most EMS textbooks are based directly on the NSC as a minimum, and many use the lessons and objectives of the NSC as the structural foundation of the text. Yet, different areas or different objectives within an area may receive more or less emphasis. It is important to consider the depth and breadth of coverage of cognitive, affective, and psychomotor content. The content must be current, relevant, and accurate. Enrichment material beyond the core content should be identified as such. The level of difficulty of the material must be consistent with the goals of the program. For example, an ALS textbook with very in-depth pathophysiology may be appropriate for paramedic students but not for intermediate students.

Paragraph 2

The content should be introduced in a table of contents. The structure of the content should be clarified through the use of chapter titles (instead of just numbers), headings, subheadings, introductions, and summaries or conclusions. Each chapter should state the objectives to be learned and provide an overview of the content. Key words should be introduced in bold type. There should be sufficient room in the margins, or "white space," to improve readability. Finally, the content must be arranged in "chunks" of suitable size so that the student can reflect upon material incrementally.

Paragraph 3

Other learning and teaching resources are available from a number of sources. Often a discussion with a medical librarian or an Internet search will help identify print or multimedia materials for which you are looking. Publishers now offer a variety of electronic and Internet-based interactive learning programs to which your program or your students may subscribe or purchase. These are generally advertised on the publisher's Web page.

Paragraph 1 Analysis

Number of sentences:	7
Total number of words:	116
Words with more than three syllables:	28
Average sentence length:	116/7 = 16.5 words
% of words with three or more syllables:	28/116 = 24%
Avg. sentence length + % of words with three or more syllables:	16.5 + 24 = 40.5
Multiply by 0.4:	40.5 × 0.4 = 16.2

Figure 15-1
(Continued)

Paragraph 2 Analysis

Number of sentences:	6
Total number of words:	93
Words with more than three syllables:	13
Average sentence length:	93/6 = 15.5
% of words with three or more syllables:	13/93 = 14%
Avg. sentence length + % of words with three or more syllables:	15.5 + 14 = 29.5
Multiply by 0.4:	$29.5 \times 0.4 = 11.8$

Paragraph 3 Analysis

Number of sentences:	4
Total number of words:	67
Words with more than three syllables:	12
Average sentence length:	67/4 = 16.8
% of words with three or more syllables:	12/67 = 18%
Avg. sentence length + % of words with three or more syllables:	16.8 + 18 = 34.8
Multiply by 0.4:	$34.8 \times 0.4 = 14$

Summary Analysis

Paragraph 1 reading level:	16.2
Paragraph 2 reading level:	11.8
Paragraph 3 reading level:	14.0
Sum:	42.0
Average:	42/3 = 14

The average reading level of the three passages is 14, which is equivalent to the reading level of a 2nd-year college student.

Note: This example is for demonstration purposes. A greater number of random passages would need to be used to get a more representative idea of the reading level.

Learning activities or review questions can be quite effective in reinforcing the text if they are relevant and properly designed. They should be of a variety of types to allow the learner choices of activities and should focus on transfer of learning rather than regurgitation of the chapter contents. If scenarios are used, they should be realistic and challenging, but solvable. All learning activities must have clear instructions.

Selection of Training Equipment and Supplies

Quantity of Supplies and Equipment

The quantity of items you will need depends upon the size and number of classes for which you will use the supplies and equipment. As a guideline, a lab group should have no greater than a 1:5 instructor-to-student ratio. You also need to consider whether multiple classes are meeting in different locations and whether or not it is feasible to share equipment between two sites. Some items need to be replenished or replaced on a regular basis, whereas others need to be budgeted less often. Your state EMS training office may have guidelines for the types and amounts of equipment and supplies your training program is required to have.

Types of Supplies and Equipment

There are a variety of equipment and supply manufacturers and vendors. You want to make sure that you are dealing with a reputable company. In addition, your institution may have established vendors that it uses and that you will be required to use. In selecting the types of equipment and supplies to be used, it is important that they are representative of what is in current use in the industry. Your training program should not use outdated types of cervical collars, splints, immobilization devices, AEDs, monitor-defibrillators, IV catheters, etc. Students have great difficulty in transferring the skills learned in the lab to the clinical setting if the equipment and supplies they will be using are greatly dissimilar. Sometimes, the use of dissimilar equipment is unavoidable. If students are doing clinical and field rotations with different agencies and institutions, each one may use different materials. In this case, it is beneficial to have a representative sample of the supplies and equipment used. This is also important if your students will be doing their certifying or registry practical examinations in an institution in which the supplies and equipment may be different than the ones used in the lab or clinical setting.

ON TARGET

It is critical to use contemporary equipment in your training program.

When selecting simulators and mannequins, the expense can easily exceed the utility of the item. It is important to look for durability, versatility, realism, cost, warranty, and availability of service. It is critical that electronic equipment, such as monitors and defibrillators, receive preventive maintenance and that it be serviced if malfunctioning. Mannequins and simulation devices must be kept in good repair. It does little good for a student to practice endotracheal intubation on a mannequin whose airway landmarks are destroyed or to practice IVs on a mannequin arm without distinguishable vasculature.

PEARLS Realism and versatility of equipment are often more important than the sophistication of the technology. High-tech simulations are appropriate when they are the only opportunity students will have to practice complicated or high-risk skills and there is no other suitable means for providing training.

Audiovisual Adjuncts

Just as a textbook is not a curriculum or course outline, neither is a PowerPoint® presentation a lesson plan. Audiovisuals—slides, videos, audiotapes, etc.—are adjuncts to the lesson plan. They are methods of presenting content. Just as they can be effectively used, they can be overused or inappropriately used. Currently, the use of PowerPoint® presentations provides the instructor with a dilemma. At the same time that many learners expect such presentations, they are overused and dominate methods of providing information. It often seems hard to please an audience in which some people complain because you used a PowerPoint® presentation and others complain because you didn't. Additionally, everyone has become a PowerPoint® "expert" and is more than happy to complain about the background color, the shape of the bullets, having five lines of text instead of four, and so forth. Given this situation, it is important to know a few guidelines for the appropriate and effective use of a variety of audiovisual adjuncts. Most such adjuncts do not require, or even allow, active participation on the part of the learner, unless the designer proceeds with student involvement in mind.

ON TARGET Just as a textbook is not a curriculum or course outline, neither is a PowerPoint® presentation a lesson plan.

PowerPoint® Presentations

PowerPoint® presentations may be a part of the instructor resource package your program has purchased or may be instructor designed. In either case, there are a few guidelines to consider. When projecting the

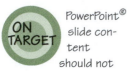

slides, as opposed to making overhead transparencies from them, it is best to use a dark background with light-colored text. Serif fonts are easier to read than sans serif fonts. For example, Times New Roman and Courier are serif fonts, whereas Arial is a sans serif font. Although it is important that the amount of text on a slide be kept to approximately five or fewer lines, also consider the importance of keeping concepts and ideas intact rather than splitting them into two slides. The integrity of the idea may be lost if the text is discontinuous. The slides should not be a word-for-word script for your presentation but should serve as a guide to important points. As with written materials, make sure that there is a point to graphics used.

Students also expect to receive the PowerPoint® slides as a handout. There are advantages and disadvantages to this. On the positive side, it provides a frame of reference and some structure for the student. On the negative side, if students already have the notes in front of them, they are less inclined to listen to and process the information you are providing orally. One solution is to save a second copy of your presentation and make modifications to it to use it as a suitable student handout. The key is to provide a bare-bones structure for students to follow, necessitating they listen and take notes to fill in missing information as you speak. However, be warned—some students will feel as if you have cheated them because you have not provided them with a copy of your presentation. This is not the case at all. It has simply become a poor practice to which students have not only become accustomed, but often consider their "right" as students. This is not conducive to student learning and you should not submit to such pressure.

Finally, a common practice of publishers is to provide a PowerPoint® slide set as an instructor resource. Although these can be quite helpful, they should not simply be an abridged edition of the text chapter. Often the same text, tables, illustrations, and photographs as those in the text are used. The purpose of the text is to prepare the student for classroom activities. No text can contain all the pertinent information students need to know. Nor can it provide the kinds of activities students need to process the information. Therefore, classroom time is not well spent by projecting onto a screen what the student should already have read. In fact, if the student comes to learn that the condensed version of his or her reading will be presented in class, they may wonder why they should do the reading outside of class at all. On the other hand, if all the student is going to get in class is what he or she already read in his text, why come to class? Of course, any presentations you construct should not mimic the text, either. Your presentation should be used to reinforce, clarify, and summarize important points, but the focus should be on showing the student how the text information can be applied.

In recent years, overhead transparencies, where still used, are often created from PowerPoint® slides. In this case, the slide background should be light or, preferably, clear, and the text should be dark. Otherwise, the same principles as those discussed for digitally projected presentations apply. Overhead projectors can also be used as a modified way of giving a "chalk talk." Instead of using a marker board or chalkboard, the speaker can write notes onto a scrolling sheet of transparency. The markers used for this purpose should be medium point with darker colors of ink. Markers are available with both erasable and permanent inks.

Marker Boards and Chalkboards

Marker boards and chalkboards are great for supporting spontaneous explanations and illustrating answers to students' questions. They also function well for teaching calculations and keeping track of questions asked and answered in case studies and scenarios. The keys are to use dark ink colors on whiteboards and light chalk colors on chalkboards and to write legibly and in large-enough letters for students to see.

 PEARLS Although they have been around for many years, marker boards and chalkboards are still great for spontaneous and dynamic activities.

Videos

Videos, as with other "easy" methods of teaching, can be overused. The cardinal rule of showing videos to your class is: Never show a video you haven't thoroughly previewed. Videos can also become outdated quickly, depending on the topic. The most important uses of video in the classroom are when you want students to see a standardized performance of a skill and in cases of last-minute instructor absences. The advantage of using a video to demonstrate skills is that, assuming the skill is demonstrated correctly in the video, the actors have the opportunity to go through many takes until they get the performance right, but the viewer only sees the right way. Often, live skill demonstrations may skip over a step or an important explanation and have to back up, causing students to become confused over the skill sequence. Videos are also good for teaching anatomy and physiology and pathophysiology when it is not feasible for students to attend a cadaver lab, view an autopsy, or see a surgical procedure. When a high-quality video is available on the appropriate topic, it is often more preferable to show the video when an instructor cancels at the last minute than it is to cancel or reschedule the class.

ON TARGET *Never show a video to your class that you have not previewed.*

Audiotapes and Computer Audio Files

The use of audiotapes and computerized audio is an especially effective way to share with class sounds that can normally be heard by only one person at a time—and then only if the proper clinical opportunity arises. The most obvious uses are for heart sounds and lung sounds. Simply describing the sounds or trying to depict them visually is inadequate and leaves a lot of room for misinterpretation. "Knowing" a sound escapes linguistic consciousness. We simply don't have the vocabulary to adequately describe most sounds. The best way to learn sounds is to hear them and have them identified in association with their description—"rales," "wheezes," etc. Otherwise, we leave the appreciation of these sounds to chance, hoping that the student will encounter the range of abnormal and normal sounds needed and that a preceptor who can help him or her identify the sounds is available.

Other Resources

Other learning and teaching resources are available from a number of sources. Often a discussion with a medical librarian or an Internet search will help identify print or multimedia materials for which you are looking. Publishers now offer a variety of electronic and Internet-based interactive learning programs to which your program or your students may subscribe or purchase. These are generally advertised on the publisher's Web page.

Summary

The wide availability of instructional materials, equipment, supplies, and methods of presentation can be overwhelming. This chapter has provided, although not a comprehensive list, a few guidelines for selecting and using instructional adjuncts. The purpose of such adjuncts is to assist the student in learning the knowledge and skills in the curriculum. Such materials must be high quality, accurate, readable, current, and well organized. They must actively engage the student to the extent possible. The role of each adjunct must be understood so that it is employed when appropriate and overuse is avoided. Such materials are often costly, and consideration must be given to the reputation of the manufacturer and vendor. Equipment must be evaluated for durability and versatility. Mannequins and simulators must be maintained in order to represent the anatomical and physiological parameters they portray accurately and realistically. All training equipment and material must be maintained in proper working order.

REVIEW QUESTIONS

1. Discuss some of the considerations in making a textbook adoption for your course.

2. What are some of the considerations in purchasing supplies and equipment for your program?

3. Give examples of when the use of a video is beneficial.

4. What are some general guidelines in creating a PowerPoint® presentation?

5. Discuss the use of lecture notes as a class handout.

16

Lesson
Planning

Learning Objectives

Upon completion of this chapter you should be able to

- Describe the importance of using a lesson plan in teaching.

- Discuss the essential components of a lesson plan.

- Differentiate between a lesson plan and a lecture outline.

- Construct an effective lesson plan for an EMS class session.

CASE
Study_____

Manuel Ibarra has been an instructor in the Harrison County Fire Department Training Academy for 3 years. He typically teaches the cardiology and medical emergencies portions of both BLS and ALS classes. One of Manny's colleagues has just been hospitalized with a myocardial infarction and will not be able to return to teaching for several weeks. Although he does not have much experience teaching trauma topics, Manny will be filling in for his colleague to teach the trauma section of an EMT-Intermediate course.

Questions

1. Should Manny use his colleague's lesson plans, use commercial lesson plans, or create his own lesson plans?
2. Given his unfamiliarity with teaching trauma, how might Manny create or modify lesson plans to effectively teach trauma topics?

Introduction

Any organized endeavor requires a plan. Teaching is no exception. The skillful organization and presentation of content and learning activities is essential to teaching effectiveness. A written lesson plan is a guide to staying on track and ensuring that all important points in a lesson are covered. A lesson plan provides additional information for the instructor, including student activities, points of emphasis, questions for critical thinking, a timeline or schedule for the session, and a list of materials needed. Lesson plans can either be created from scratch or adapted from commercially prepared packages. In this chapter, you will learn about the usefulness of lesson plans and the essential components that should be included in a lesson plan, whether you create it yourself or adapt it from another instructor or commercial package.

What Is a Lesson Plan?

 A lesson plan is a map, blueprint, or guide for the instructor to use in successfully navigating through the class session.

A lesson plan is not simply a lecture, discussion outline, or PowerPoint® presentation. It provides information about the context and timing of the lesson, what types of teaching-learning activities will be used, the equipment, supplies, and other resources needed, a list of references for the content of the lesson, and other important information. For example, some lesson plans include a place to note class announcements and administrative items. A lesson plan can be thought of as a map, a blueprint, or guide for the instructor to use in successfully navigating through the class session.

Lesson plans are important for a number of reasons. They function as a guide to organizing the lesson and keeping it on track. Lesson plans provide the instructor with not only the content of the lesson, but also a plan for preparing for, conducting, and evaluating the class session. A prepared lesson plan may be useful when an instructor needs to step in at the last moment to teach a class, but there are drawbacks to picking up a lesson plan prepared by someone else. A lesson plan is not a script for a lecture. Unless the instructor is already knowledgeable in the topic being presented, the lesson plan will be of little value. Additionally, each instructor has his or her own preferences for what is included in a lesson plan and how much detail it provides. On this same note, a lesson plan should be a work in progress, never a completed document. Lesson plans must be reviewed and updated each time they are used, not simply dusted off and used again.

A preprepared lesson plan may be useful, but it still requires preparation on the part of the classroom instructor.

Components of a Lesson Plan

There are various formats for lesson plans. They usually consist of a heading area with the title of the lesson, a description of the audience, the date, the name of the instructor, equipment and supplies needed, references, a list of student handouts, and the amount of time needed for the lesson. The lesson plan contains a list of the objectives to be accomplished through the content and activities included in the plan. The body of the lesson plan is typically divided into columns. Depending on your preference and style, you may wish to use the page in landscape (sidewise) orientation rather than portrait (upright) orientation. Column headings may include the time, the main topic, teaching points, media or audiovisuals, and instructor notes. At the end of the lesson plan, you may include an area for notes to remind yourself of changes you want to make to the lesson plan before using it again. Figure 16-1 provides an example of a lesson plan. You may prefer to use a lesson plan that is more detailed than the one shown.

PEARLS Lesson plans must be faithful to principles of instruction but should be tailored to your needs and preferences as an instructor.

Constructing a Lesson Plan

In order to construct a lesson plan, you need to know several things. Foremost among these are an understanding of the audience, the objectives for the lesson, and the time allotted for the lesson. Understanding the audience includes knowing what their prior experiences entail so that you can anticipate what the participants already know and their perspective on a given topic, as well as the depth and breadth of content required to meet their needs. Understanding the audience also provides input into the selection of teaching-learning activities for the lesson. Knowing the objectives is critical to providing the structure and content of the lesson, as well as selecting the appropriate methods for teaching the content. Finally, the time allowed will help you make decisions about activities and prioritize content.

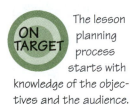

The lesson planning process starts with knowledge of the objectives and the audience.

Providing the content of the lesson plan begins with research based on the objectives. You should begin with the students' textbook, but you should also consult supplementary texts, journal articles, and perhaps experts and other sources of information. At the beginning of the research process, you should include in your notes as many ideas as you think are relevant. You can narrow these ideas down later in the process.

Figure 16-1
Lesson Plan

Date:_____	Time_____ Location:_____ Instructor:_____
Module:	Paramedic National Standard Curriculum Module 1—Preparatory
Lesson:	Medication Administration
Time:	1-hour lecture, 3-hour lab
Student Preparation:	Read text Chapter 10 and the medication administration skills section of the course laboratory manual.
Student Prerequisites:	Completion of general pharmacology and mathematics for drug-dosage calculation.
Instructor Prep:	Review task analyses for medication administration skills and review student reading.
Asst. Instructors:	Mark, Jeff, Jaime
Methods:	Lecture-discussion, demonstration, guided skills practice
EMS Equipment and Supplies Needed:	Alcohol preps, bandaids, IV dressings, 1-in. and 2-in. tape, 4-in. $\times$ 4-in. gauze squares, gloves, various sizes of needles, IV catheters, and syringes; IV tubing, IV fluid, IV poles, vials of sterile water or saline, selection of medications in vials and prefilled syringes, IV mannequin arms, disposable absorbent underpads, oranges, medication cups, water cups, small candies, biohazard disposal containers, clipboards, patient care forms.
AV Equipment:	Digital projector, laptop computer, presentation CD, VCR/TV and medication skills video.
Special Arrangements:	Will need four lab rooms.
Administrative Items and Announcements:	Attendance sign-in sheet. Collect homework assignment 2.
	Assign homework 3.
	Reminder that clinical paperwork must be handed in on time.

Objectives

By the end of this lesson the student should be able to:

Cognitive

01. Describe the enteral and parenteral routes of medication administration.

02. Identify the equipment and supplies needed to administer medications by each route.

03. Discuss the advantages and disadvantages of medication administration via each route.

04. Describe the techniques used in the administration of medication by each route.

05. Identify anatomy and physiology related to the administration of medications by each route.

06. Explain the legal aspects of medication administration.

07. Given a scenario, collect all information needed to ensure safe, effective medication administration.

08. Explain what patient assessment parameters must be reassessed after administering medications.

Affective

01. Advocate the use of body-substance isolation as needed in the administration of medication.

02. Value the importance of proper disposal of contaminated sharps.

03. Value the criticality of careful delivery of service in the administration of medications.

04. Defend the importance of careful documentation of medication administration.

Psychomotor

01. Given a scenario, prepare a medication ordered for administration by each route.

02. Given a scenario, demonstrate the administration of medication by each route.

03. Demonstrate the safe use and disposal of equipment and supplies used for administering medications.

Time	Content/Activities	Notes	Media
0800	Overview	Review objectives	Slides 1–5
	Principles of medication		
	Administration and the "six rights"	Tell story about lidocaine overdose at General Hospital.	Slides 6–8
	• Importance of repeating back orders		Slide 9
	Medical direction		
	• Online		
	• Off-line		
	BSI and equipment disposal	Talk about the preceptor who always stuck used needles into the foam mattress of the cot.	Slides 10, 11
	• Never recap!		
	Medical asepsis: sterile, aseptic, clean, disinfection. Describe importance of friction and use of concentric circles in site preparation.		Slides 12–15

Figure 16-1
(Continued)

Time	Content/Activities	Notes	Media
0820	Routes of administration: Indications, contraindications, advantages, and disadvantages • Percutaneous • Transdermal • Mucus membranes • Pulmonary • Enteral • Parenteral • Injections sites • Key points of technique	Include endotracheal administration—"NAVEL." Ask students to describe each of the different forms of enteral medications. Describe packaging, syringes, needles, IV tubing.	Slides 16–22
0850	Documentation Summary		Slide 23 Slides 24, 25
0900	Break		
0910	Lab groups: 4 groups of 4 students each		
	For each skill: • Instructors introduce skill. • Instructors demonstrate total activity. • Demonstrate step-by-step with explanation. • Instructors demonstrate total activity. • Students practice with feedback. • Instructors debrief and summarize.	Breaks as needed. Students assist with cleanup.	Student skill sheets
1200	Dismissal		

Student evaluation: 10-point quiz on medication administration next class session

Lesson/instructor evaluation: Debrief lab instructors

Lesson revision: Elaborate more on advantages and disadvantages of each route of administration

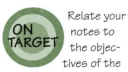

Relate your notes to the objectives of the lesson so you can sequence the material and ensure coverage of the objectives.

Be sure that you relate material to the objectives of the lesson so you can later sequence the material and so that you can be sure that you have covered all the objectives you intended to.

Next you should sequence the content for effectiveness. The lesson plan begins by making a connection with prior knowledge and experience. You should then consider principles of learning in constructing the sequence of content and activities. The material should proceed from what is known to what is unknown and from simple to complex. The order of the information must be logical. At this point, you can begin to eliminate, or perhaps add, content based on its quantity and quality.

It will take some time before you become accustomed to how much material can be covered using particular teaching methods in a given amount of time. New instructors often over- or underestimate the amount of material that can be covered. It is very helpful to include a column for time in the lesson plan in order to pace yourself. You might also give consideration to having supplemental activities as a backup in the event that your lesson runs much shorter than expected. If you find yourself ahead of schedule, you can slow down and allow for more questions and discussion. If you find yourself behind schedule, you can make adjustments on the fly, making sure you hit the most important points and perhaps reducing the amount of elaboration and discussion.

 Have a backup plan of supplemental activities in case your content doesn't fill the time period.

Using a Lesson Plan

The point of having students sit in a classroom is to provide them with an effective educational experience. In order to achieve this, the session must be planned, and the plan must be followed. Many speakers, although highly personable or entertaining, fail to use a lesson plan in favor of extemporaneous speaking and delivering anecdotes about their field experiences. Because there is no plan to cover the objectives, the objectives are usually not covered, and students are denied the opportunity to receive instruction. Occasionally, an instructor comes into the classroom with a lesson plan but is sidetracked from it, so the entire lesson gets derailed. Many instructors feel there is some weakness in relying on a lesson plan or lecture notes. This is not the case at all. No one can remember an entire lesson in its proper sequence. The lesson plan is an instructional tool used to keep the lesson on track. The goal is to provide the students with a complete and organized learning activity.

PEARLS *The point of creating a lesson plan is to use it in the classroom.*

The use of a lesson plan prepared by another instructor or one that is part of an instructor resource package, although convenient, may have some drawbacks. In using these materials, there is a temptation to underprepare for the lesson by skipping the research step. The lesson plan may not suit your style, or it may need to be modified to meet your needs. In using such materials, it is critical that you review the lesson plan well ahead of the class session to make sure that it contains all the elements you need to teach your class and that you are thoroughly familiar with the content to be delivered and the methods by which it will be delivered.

Summary

Lesson planning is a critical step in the instructional process, but it is often skipped for a variety of reasons. Lesson plans contain crucial information about the content, sequence, timing, and methods of instruction. Although lesson planning can be an arduous process, particularly for new instructors, it is a step that cannot be omitted in the delivery of quality education. With practice, you will learn to adapt lesson plans to your own style and needs.

REVIEW QUESTIONS

1. Discuss the purposes of creating and using lesson plans.

2. Discuss the key components of a lesson plan.

3. What information is needed in order to construct a lesson plan?

4. Describe the general process for developing a lesson plan.

Methods
of Instruction

Upon completion of this chapter you should be able to

- Compare and contrast methods of instruction in terms of their uses, advantages, and disadvantages.

- Given a description of class learning needs, select an appropriate instructional method for accomplishing the intended learning outcomes.

- Prepare notes for lectures and discussions.

- Relate principles of effective communication to the teaching-learning transaction.

- Deliver an effective presentation.

- Utilize questions to facilitate discussion.

- Discuss principles of using written papers, projects, and assignments as a student learning activity.

- Discuss the appropriate use of games and case-based teaching.

- Describe the essential features of computer-based instruction.

CASE Study

Latrice Wallace is doing a teaching internship with the Gaddis Township Vocational School. Because she is an EMT, she has been assigned to the health careers section to assist with the EMT class. She has been asked to present a lesson on geriatrics. The students in the EMT class are either high school seniors in the health careers program or are adult students who have been referred through vocational counseling, because they are currently unemployed or want to change careers.

Questions

1. What teaching-learning methods might be appropriate for this task?
2. What questions could Latrice use to stimulate discussion?
3. Are there any activities you might recommend that Latrice avoid?
4. Because Latrice is an inexperienced instructor, what can she do to decrease her anxiety about her teaching assignment?

Introduction

Traditionally, texts on teaching talk about methods of teaching. What goes on in the classroom, however, is more about student learning. Of course, the instructor has a vital role to play, but it is important to think of classroom activity as a transaction between the instructor and learner in order to recognize that learning is an active process and that the learner must be engaged in it. The more learner centered the method, the more active the learner will be. There are a number of considerations in selecting a method for the **teaching-learning transaction.** Some of these considerations include class size, objectives to be achieved, time allotted for the lesson, space and equipment available, availability of adjunct instructors, cost, and at what point students are in a particular program. Regardless of the method selected, effective communication is of the essence. In this chapter, you will learn about principles of effective classroom communication and various ways of facilitating the teaching-learning transaction.

teaching-learning transaction
A term used to convey the reciprocal roles of the teacher and learner in the educational setting.

KEY TERMS

case-based teaching, p. 267

communication, p. 268

computer-based instruction (CBI), p. 268

diction, p. 270

discussion, p. 263

dysfluencies, p. 272

facilitation, p. 272

lecture, p. 261

Instructional Techniques

Lecture

lecture
A method of instruction that relies on one-way communication from the instructor to the students.

The **lecture** remains the most commonly used, overused, and misused teaching method that exists. There are times when lecture is appropriate, but as a teaching-learning method, it has some drawbacks. Lectures are useful when there is a large amount of background information to be given, when there is a large audience, when the instructor wants to bring material not available in the textbook to students' attention, and when the instructor needs to maintain control of the topic. Lecturing is also an effective means of allowing for repetition of key points. However, effective lecturing is not easy. It takes considerable planning of both content and delivery. Additionally, lecture is a very passive means for students to acquire information and relies on one-way communication. Because of this, recall—and especially application—of knowledge is poor as compared to other methods. Students' processing of information delivered in lecture format is improved when they take notes, when a visual framework for organization is provided, and when it is clear that they will be called upon to summarize the information at the end of the class session.

One of the drawbacks of lectures is that it is difficult to maintain listeners' attention. We can mentally process information much more quickly than it can be spoken aloud, allowing the listener's focus to drift. Typically, attention is highest in the first 10 minutes of a lecture and declines thereafter. Using variation in the tone and volume of speech and using pauses can all serve to refocus students' attention. The use of visual aids can help but must not be a word-for-word script of the lecture. Remember, it is important for learners to take notes during lectures. Handing out copies of lecture notes is not effective if learning is the goal of the lecture. Handing out a skeleton outline of the lecture, though, can be useful in helping the learner organize his or her notes.

PEARLS Lectures are often used when other teaching-learning methods might be more effective. There is a common misperception that it is easier to lecture than it is to use other methods, but lecturing places most of the responsibility for the class session on the instructor. Allowing students to participate puts more responsibility on the students and allows them to become involved in their own learning.

Lectures must be effectively organized, using principles of learning. The sequence and organization of material is important, as is occasionally summing up the major points covered thus far. The use of examples and relating the information to learners' experiences and what they already know help to anchor the information. Using the following components of a lecture will help you plan and deliver an effective lecture.

- **Orientation:** Present information to get learners' attention and focus it on the direction of the lecture. One way in which you can orient learners to the lecture topic is to provide an anecdote or discuss a current event in which the information about to be delivered is relevant.
- **Enthusiasm:** Enthusiastic delivery conveys the importance of the topic.
- **Variety:** Using inflection, volume, gestures, movement, and AV materials helps capture the learners' attention.
- **Organization:** Logical sequencing of material helps in providing smooth transitions between topics and provides a cognitive structure to aid in retention. Deliver the material in "chewable chunks." That is, avoid information overload.
- **Explanation:** Describe and expound on facts, concepts, and principles in a clear manner.
- **Directions:** Providing instruction on how to approach a situation helps with cognitive organization and symbolic rehearsal of events.
- **Illustration:** Provide clear, relevant, interesting examples of how the information can be applied. This reinforces the importance of the material and helps in retention.
- **Comparing and contrasting:** Present the similarities and differences, advantages and disadvantages, and other features of two phenomena, interventions, etc. For example, compare and contrast congestive heart failure and COPD.
- **Questioning and discussion:** Emphasize important points and elicit feedback on student understanding.
- **Summarizing:** Highlight important concepts and link ideas together. This should be done periodically throughout the lesson, as well as at the end of the lecture, to deliver information in easily assimilated amounts.

One of the challenges of lecturing is to remember the thoughts, anecdotes, and insights you want to impart to students at the time in the lecture that they are the most effective. This brings us to the use of lecture notes. A lecture outline with notes in the margin, such as the format demonstrated in Chapter 16 for lesson plans, provides structure and organization without risking lapsing into reading the lecture verbatim.

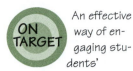

An effective way of engaging students' attention during a lecture is to let the students know you will be calling upon them to help summarize the information at the end of the session.

The typical format of a lecture is to tell them what you're going to tell them, tell them, and then tell them what you told them. That is, there should be an introduction with an overview, the body or content of the lecture, and a summary. There are benefits to this method. However, an alternative is to let the learners know ahead of time that they will be expected to summarize the lecture verbally at the end of the lesson. This motivates students to pay attention in order to avoid embarrassment later when they are called on for their summaries. It also encourages deeper processing of the information. You can also effectively deliver a summary by presenting a scenario or posing a problem for students to solve rather than by rephrasing the lecture material.

Discussion

discussion
An instructional technique that allows for meaningful verbal communication between students and the instructor.

A guided class **discussion** has the benefit of providing structure but encouraging student participation. Discussion can take place in the larger class group or in smaller groups. If small groups are used, they can report summaries of their discussions to the larger group at the end of the period.

A distinct advantage of discussion over lecture is that it gives the instructor an opportunity to evaluate student knowledge and reasoning ability. Additionally, student experiences can be drawn into the discussion, increasing the relevance of the material and encouraging students to prepare for class. Discussion can also be used to assist students in developing problem-solving skills.

 Allowing students to talk allows the instructor to evaluate their knowledge.

A discussion should begin with a problem to be solved, such as a case study, or a controversy, such as "Should paramedics be able to refuse to transport patients under particular conditions?" The instructor can provide clarification and ask questions to stimulate student thinking about the problem. Playing devil's advocate is also a way to stimulate student thinking. As an instructor, you should record the relevant points of the discussion for visual reference and occasionally pause to summarize the discussion. You must keep the discussion on track if it starts to stray and mediate disagreements among group members. See Box 17-1 for a list of guidelines for asking questions, Box 17-2 for a list of discussion-facilitating questions, Box 17-3 for types of questions, and Box 17-4 for suggested responses for keeping the discussion on track.

Guidelines for Asking Questions

- Provide a frame of reference; give enough information so students can formulate a response.
- Prompt the answer if necessary, but give students a chance to answer. Try not to interrupt or answer your own question.
- Anticipate some possible answers you might get, both correct and incorrect.
- Ask specific questions; plan them ahead of time.
- Be nonjudgmental and respond in a positive way.
- Don't ask the same question more than twice—either rephrase the question or ask a series of simpler questions that lead up to the correct answer.
- Repeat the correct response. This emphasizes the correct answers, ensures that everyone heard it, and provides positive reinforcement.
- Don't rely on the same people to answer all the time.

Questions for Facilitating Discussion

Clarifying Responses

- Can you give me an example?
- What do you mean by _____?
- If you did that, where would it lead? What would be the consequences?
- Are you saying that . . .? (Either restate the correct answer, or distort the answer to get the student to clarify.)
- What assumptions would we have to make for things to work out that way? (This forces students to look at the bigger picture.)
- What are some other possibilities?
- How do you know that's right?
- Is that consistent with what you know about _____?

Box 17-3

Types of Questions

Direct: Aimed at one person.

- "Dennis, what is the first action you would take at this scene?"

Indirect: Thrown out to the group.

- If no one answers, look for nonverbal clues that someone may have the answer and call on him or her.

Factual (convergent): One correct answer, doesn't keep the discussion going.

Divergent: Encourages discussion.

- "What do you think about _____?"

Double-check: Checks for student understanding.

- "So what you mean is _____?"

Assumptive: Serves as a reminder or suggestion.

- "You'd want to use a large-bore IV for that, wouldn't you?"

Summary: States the objectives in the form of questions.

Lecture-Discussion

Many classroom presentations are a hybrid between lecture and discussion. Often, beginning students do not have enough information or experience to keep a discussion going. **Lecture-discussion** involves providing information through lecture and facilitating discussion at intervals throughout the lesson to allow students to receive information and immediately have an opportunity to process it more fully.

lecture-discussion
A more interactive approach to traditional lecture that includes planned areas for group discussion.

Student Assignments as a Method of Learning

Papers, journals, reports, assignments, and projects, if designed and used properly, can be effective methods through which students can learn. Such activities must have a clear purpose based on course objectives. These types of activities stimulate active learning and introduce students to self-directed learning. With increasing emphasis on evidence-based

Box 17-4

Suggested Responses for Managing Group Interaction

Long-winded speakers:

- "You lost me. Could you summarize what you just said?"

Off-the-wall comments:

- "Can you explain how that relates to (the topic at hand)?"
- "I'm not sure I understand why you're saying that."

Silent students:

- "Dan, we haven't heard from you. What are your thoughts on this?"

Overly enthusiastic students:

- "We haven't heard from some of the others. Let's see what everyone else thinks."

Argumentative students:

- "Explain your thinking so I can understand where you're coming from."

Unresolved disagreements:

- "I don't think we're going to solve this today. Let's move on with the rest of our discussion for now."

Digression/sidetracking

- "We were talking about (topic). Let's get back to that."

---

practice, abstracting research articles can be an effective way of getting students to be critical consumers of medical literature. Such an assignment can lead to in-class presentations in which students share what they have learned with other students, creating a learning community. Depending upon the composition of your class, you may need to provide a framework for literature analysis and perhaps a couple of examples for students to review prior to such an assignment. You may also need to clarify what you consider to be acceptable sources of literature and how students can access those sources.

When assigning papers, it is important to be clear about the topic, structure, and length of the paper. Let students know what referencing format you will accept and give them information on where to find the guidelines for that format. Make it clear that plagiarism is cheating and will not be tolerated. Unfortunately, with the phenomenal amount of information available electronically, there is a huge increase in instances of copying and pasting materials into papers and assignments. This offense is often difficult and time consuming to prove. From experience, some of the things that have given students away are including hyperlinks in the text, the use of British or Canadian spellings or phrases by students not from those countries, and the use of a writing style that is inconsistent with the student's previously demonstrated style. One way of reducing the likelihood of plagiarism is to request that students submit their assignments in their own handwriting.

 PEARLS You may want to invite a speaker from a college or university writing lab to provide your students with tips on researching and writing papers.

Case-based Teaching

case-based teaching
A versatile method of instruction that puts problems to be presented to students in context.

Case-based teaching is an excellent method for establishing for students their need to know in a manner that creates curiosity. Presenting a case at the beginning of class and posing questions about it clues learners in to the importance of the material being covered to the problem at hand. In essence, learners are motivated to learn because what they currently know is insufficient to solve the problem presented. Cases can also be used for reinforcement, critical thinking, and review exercises. Commercially produced cases can be somewhat expensive but generally have the advantage of saving the instructor time in preparation and providing the questions for discussion, answers, and further references.

The alternative is to create your own cases based on real-life situations. Of course, these cases must not reveal any information that can lead to identification of the patient. It is important to provide enough information to frame the situation, but to omit details that could only be elicited through the history and physical exam so that the students learn to seek the appropriate information. Cases can be discussed as a class or by dividing students into small groups. Cases can also be assigned to individuals or groups as homework assignments or presentations.

Instructional Games

Games can provide variety and fun in the classroom but should be used only if they accomplish a clear educational objective. You can find ideas and materials for games in instructor resource kits accompanying textbooks, or you can create your own. You may find it worthwhile to invest in the series *Games Trainers Play* (Scannell and Newstrom, McGraw-Hill) as a source of ideas for productive games. You can also create EMS versions of popular television game shows such as *Jeopardy* and the *$10,000 Pyramid*. Games tend to be most useful for reinforcement and review rather than for providing information.

Computer-based Instruction

computer-based instruction (CBI) The use of software or Internet platform–based programs to deliver instructional content, engage students in activities, and allow communication between students and the instructor.

Computer-based instruction (CBI) is becoming more prevalent all the time. Instructional programs may be available online or as software packages or can be created by the instructor using a Web platform such as Blackboard™ or WebCT™. CBI can be used for distance education for students who never enter your classroom or as an adjunct to traditional classroom activities. Well-designed CBI is interactive, gives the learner feedback, and suggests a pace for the learner to follow. There are principles guiding the effective design of CBI programs, as well as for effectively managing a distance education course, although it is beyond the scope of this text to provide these guidelines. If you plan to use CBI, it is recommended that you take a course in instructional design systems or distance education.

Presentation and Facilitation Skills
Communication

communication The exchange of meaning between two or more parties by any effective means.

Communication is the mutual exchange of information between parties by any effective means. As an instructor, you communicate with students in a variety of ways. You use speaking, writing, demonstrations, and more subtle forms of communication, such as the way you dress and interact with students. You will find yourself in the roles of both sender and receiver in the communication process.

 PEARLS You are always communicating something, whether you realize it or not.

The Sender Role

sender The individual from whom a message originates.

As the **sender,** an instructor must take care to communicate effectively. In previous writing, communications, or English classes you may have learned that to send an effective message you must consider *who, what, when, where,* and *how.* We concern ourselves here mostly with the *who, what, when,* and *how.* You must begin with a thorough understanding of the material you are going to present. This is the *what* of your message. You must determine what is relevant for your audience and how much detail and background information are needed to make the message understandable.

To effectively communicate your understanding, you must understand *who* your audience is. What is their prior experience? Is English their native language? *Why* is the information important for this audience? How is it relevant to them? What learner needs does the information satisfy? Timing of the message is vital. *When* should this information be delivered? Information is best understood in context and in the appropriate sequence. Has the appropriate prerequisite material been covered? Will the learners have a timely opportunity to use the information? Finally, you must choose *how* you are going to deliver the message.

The Receiver Role

receiver
The individual to whom a message is delivered.

As an instructor you must be a **receiver**—that is, you must receive messages from the class participants, as well. You must strive not only to be a good listener, but also to seek out feedback from learners to assess their understanding. You must also look for the puzzled facial expressions, looks of boredom, and the restlessness that may signal the need to take a break. To check your understanding of the message, demonstrate active listening responses, such as paraphrasing the speaker's words. Concentrate on what is being said. This is much more easily said than done. We can process information at a much faster rate than we can speak. Therefore, our thoughts often race ahead of what the speaker is saying, and we lose part of the message. We also sometimes let our personal interests and emotions get in our way of listening to a message.

Barriers to Communication

There is a variety of factors that can interfere with communication. Language, as will be discussed shortly, emotions of the sender or receiver, nonverbal language, preconceived notions, assumptions, and jumping to conclusions can all interfere with communication. It is often what we think we know that keeps us from listening to the message of another.

The Use of Language and Grammar in Communication

semantics
The meaning of language.

English can be a complicated language to understand because the most common English words generally have multiple meanings. We also have a variety of vocabulary choices in phrasing our messages. **Semantics,** the interpreted meaning of words, can be an issue in understanding, as can tone or voice inflection. Messages should not contain more words than necessary to impart meaning. We are all familiar with speakers who go on and on, either repeating the same message or, perhaps, never getting to the message. Given our speed of thought versus the speed of speech, an overly wordy speaker is going to lose the audience to their own thoughts. Another issue in language is the use of slang, jargon, and unnecessarily complex vocabulary. Remember, language is for expression, not impression. Why refer to your gas tank as a fuel-containment module or your cellular phone as a portable, personal two-way communication device when simple language is so much more effective?

 PEARLS Tape-record a lecture or two to get an idea of your verbal communication style. We are often unconscious of many of our verbal idiosyncrasies.

diction
Degree of clarity and distinctness of pronunciation in speech.

Poor grammar, punctuation, and **diction** (articulation, pronunciation, and projection of speech) also interfere with communication. In written communication, poor spelling is a barrier to understanding. Although spell-checking programs can help in word-processed documents, a misspelling of a word that results in the formation of another, correctly spelled word will not be caught. Neither will using *principle* instead of *principal* or *effective* instead of *affective*. Unless you have installed a medical terminology spell-checking program on your computer, you will need to pay particular attention to the spelling of medical terms. Proofreading is essential. Unfortunately, neither spell checking or proofreading are options when you are writing on a marker board or blackboard.

General Considerations in Classroom Teaching

Whether you are leading a discussion or presenting information, there are some common tasks that will increase your effectiveness and sense of ease. Begin by paying attention to the classroom environment and climate. The physical arrangement must be conducive to your purposes. Seating should be arranged so that learners have a clear view of the presenter and any audiovisuals to be used. For discussion, they should preferably have a clear view of each other, as well.

Practice with your AVs. Project your slides before the day of the presentation to ensure that your computer is compatible with the projector provided and that the slides are easily read from even the back of the classroom. Try to secure a room that is free of distractions, such as noise, flickering overhead lights, and extremes of temperature. Seating should be comfortable so that attention is not drawn from the presentation or discussion to the sensation of physical discomfort.

Set the tone of the class by arriving early and speaking to participants as they arrive. This will put both you and them at ease. By doing this with an unfamiliar audience, you will have a few friendly faces in the crowd when you begin your presentation. Although it is most certainly not necessary to be an entertainer (or edutainer, as it is sometimes called), nor should it be expected of you, the use of natural, appropriate humor goes a long way toward setting both the speaker and the audience at ease. It is important that you are able to laugh at yourself and that any humor you use is not at the expense of an individual or group.

It is important to establish your credibility as an instructor. If you are greeting a class for the first time, it is important to provide them with an overview of your educational preparation and experience in the area about which you are speaking. Your audience should know what qualifies you to speak on a particular subject. It is equally important, though, that you don't go overboard and give the impression that you are full of yourself. Establish your credibility on your own merits and avoid name dropping and listing all the activities in which you have been involved in an attempt to establish your qualifications.

Quelling Your Anxiety

For most people unaccustomed to public speaking, the prospect of talking in front of a group can be quite overwhelming. In fact, by some accounts, fear of public speaking is rated the number one fear that people have, rating higher than even fear of snakes or heights. The good news is that not only are there ways to reduce your anxiety, but to some degree you can actually use your anxiety to energize your presentation.

One of the keys to reducing the anxiety associated with public speaking is to prepare. A thoroughly prepared and practiced presentation gives you a sense of competence and confidence. Arrive early, become acclimated to the facility, and meet some of the participants. Keep a noncaffeinated beverage nearby. Anxiety causes thirst, and thirst makes speaking difficult. Anxiety also often results in rapid speech, so taking a sip of water here and there will help slow you down. If you are nervous about speaking, avoid caffeine prior to and during your presentation, because it will exacerbate your anxiety and the symptoms it produces.

Physical movement helps reduce anxiety by utilizing the stress response to your advantage.

ON TARGET

Anxiety stimulates the release of catecholamines and mobilizes you for action. A little stress or anxiety actually improves performance, but beyond a certain amount it is detrimental to performance. Moving about rather than anchoring yourself behind the podium will help utilize this excess energy. Just be certain that your moving about is purposeful, not distracting to the learners.

It is helpful in both reducing anxiety and refining your presentation skills to videotape, or at least audiotape, yourself as you practice your

Box 17-5

Contrasting Teacher and Facilitator

Teacher	Facilitator
Presents information	Guides discussion
Provides the right answers	Provides the right questions
One-way communication	Two-way communication
Gives assignments	Coordinates learning activities
Dictates objectives	Incorporates group's relevant goals
Teacher-centered	Learner-centered

dysfluencies
Utterances of habit such as um, ah, you know, you see, etc., that are spoken frequently and almost unconsciously and interfere with the articulation of a spoken message.

facilitation
The use of enabling statements, questions, and nonverbal communication to manage productive classroom discussion.

presentation. At the very least, ask a trusted mentor to observe you and give you feedback on your performance. Some of the qualities of your presentation you will want to monitor include dysfluencies, volume, rate of speech, and physical habits. **Dysfluencies** are utterances of habit such as um, ah, you know, you see, etc., that are spoken frequently and almost unconsciously and interfere with the articulation of a spoken message.

Facilitation

As an instructor you will both teach and facilitate learning. These two activities are different, as illustrated in Box 17-5. **Facilitation** offers a number of benefits in the teaching-learning transaction. Students are allowed the opportunity to express their views and opinions, there is an opportunity to foster respect for others' perspectives, students have the opportunity to improve their verbal communication skills, students take ownership for information, and facilitated discussion is participative and can be fun. A fundamental part of facilitating learning is asking the right questions and managing the group interaction. Guidelines for these tasks are listed in Boxes 17-1, 17-2, and 17-4.

Summary

Basic knowledge of the uses, advantages, and disadvantages of various instructional methods will help you select the most effective means of meeting particular instructional objectives. The essence of all the methods discussed is effective communication. There are a number of steps you can take to ensure a quality presentation or discussion. These are skills that develop over time, so don't give up if your first few attempts at teaching don't go as well as you had hoped. In this chapter we discussed cognitive teaching methods. In Chapter 19 we discuss effective methods of clinical and laboratory instruction.

REVIEW QUESTIONS

1. Describe ways to increase the effectiveness of lectures.

2. What are the benefits of discussion as a method of instruction?

3. What is one of the primary advantages of using student assignments as a method of learning?

4. Discuss considerations in case-based teaching.

5. What is the most appropriate use of games in the classroom?

6. What are some of the characteristics of effective computer-based instruction (CBI)?

7. What are some common barriers to effective communication?

8. Discuss tips for reducing your anxiety as a classroom instructor.

9. Discuss benefits of facilitation in the teaching-learning transaction.

Classroom
Management

Learning Objectives

Upon completion of this chapter you should be able to

- Describe the characteristics of a positive learning environment.

- Identify dysfunctional student behaviors.

- Given a description of a learning environment issue, formulate a plan for approaching the problem.

- Role-model positive classroom behaviors.

- Describe measures to maintain group order and productivity.

- Discuss means for encouraging student participation.

- Relate theories of motivation to student behavior.

- Discuss means for handling specific dysfunctional student behaviors.

- Identify barriers to student motivation.

- Discuss measures that can reduce or eliminate barriers to student motivation.

CASE
Study_____

Bart is 20-year-old college student taking your paramedic course, which consists of both certificate and degree-seeking students. The degree-seeking students are college-age students enrolled full time in the university. The majority of students are full-time, paid career public safety personnel who are seeking a paramedic certificate. Bart is very bright, but he is a "know-it-all" who often cannot appreciate what he does *not* know. He has been a volunteer for 6 months for a rescue squad in his hometown, in a nontransporting role. He thinks he is very experienced as a result of this. Bart is very cheerful and talks nearly incessantly. He tries very hard to look and talk the part, but he overdoes it. During lab scenarios he gets very loud and excited and becomes bossy, barking out orders rather than providing team leadership. He is condescending to his teammates, patients, and families in the scenarios, although he doesn't realize this. In fact, he is oblivious to others' reactions to his behavior. In addition, his cell phone rings frequently and he often "forgets" to turn it off during class. He often comes in several minutes late and dozes off during class. Today, while you have a guest lecturer teaching an incident command lesson, Bart is monopolizing class discussion, and his classmates are obviously annoyed by him.

Questions

1. What do you think might be motivating Bart's behaviors?
2. Why might this issue be particularly difficult to address?
3. What are some ways in which you could address Bart's behavior?

Introduction

One of your important tasks as an instructor is to manage class interactions in order to establish and maintain a positive, productive learning environment. There are a number of activities that go into this effort, but one of the most difficult is handling dysfunctional student behaviors in the classroom. Sometimes people worry about violating the rights of the student who needs to be addressed. Looking at the bigger picture, any student behaving in a manner that negatively impacts the learning environment is violating the rights of the other students. As the group leader, it is incumbent upon you to act on behalf of the group in establishing and maintaining the integrity of the learning environment. To do this, you will need a basic understanding of motivation. In this chapter you will learn about establishing a tolerant and comfortable learning environment in which students can feel safe asking and answering questions, removing barriers to student motivation, enhancing class participation, and identifying and addressing dysfunctional student behaviors.

The Learning Environment

Both the physical and emotional characteristics of the classroom are important in creating a positive, productive learning climate. Physically, students should have comfortable seating with sufficient personal space, be able to see the instructor and audiovisuals, and have a large enough table or desk space to arrange their materials. Depending upon the size of the group and the objectives of the lesson, a variety of seating arrangements can be used. Arranging tables or desks in a square or horseshoe shape facilitates discussion, because students can see each other. This arrangement also makes it more difficult for students to "hide" from the instructor by sitting in the back of the room. As an aside, you should ask yourself if you are giving students a reason to want to hide from you. Perhaps they feel uncomfortable with your reactions to their questions and comments. For small-group work, tables or desks can be moved into clusters. This makes it easy for the instructor to move from group to group to assess and assist in group processes.

ON TARGET The learning environment has both physical and psychological components.

The room temperature should be comfortable. If there is disagreement about a comfortable room temperature, setting the thermostat on the cooler side allows colder students to wear a sweater or sweatshirt without making warmer participants sleepy or inattentive due to physical discomfort. Proper lighting is also important and should be adjustable for use with projected audiovisuals.

Ideally, the classroom should be free from audible and visual distractions. Course policies and practices should address the use—or, more accurately, nonuse—of pagers and cellular phones by students. In settings where it is an issue, overhead paging and alarm systems should be turned off. If the classroom is in a busy building, you may need to keep the door closed. If heating, air-conditioning, fans, or other equipment is too noisy, it should be serviced to minimize noise.

ON TARGET Important physical characteristics of the learning environment include the temperature, room arrangement, personal space, comfort of seating, organization, freedom from distractions, and visibility of the instructor and audiovisuals.

In the laboratory setting, equipment must be in sufficient supply and acceptable condition. Attention to student safety is important, as is ensuring adequate space for laboratory activities. A neatly organized storage area, well-maintained equipment, and uncluttered workspace communicate the value of the equipment and how it should be cared for to the students.

Emotionally, students must feel secure and accepted. They must feel they can contribute to discussions, demonstrate tasks, and ask questions or attempt to answer questions without fear of ridicule or harsh criticism. This requires not only the instructor's attitude of acceptance, but also that the instructor act as a student advocate and ensure that students treat each other with respect. As an instructor, you can also play a role in the stress level of the course. A moderate amount of stress stimulates performance, but an overwhelming amount of stress detracts from performance. Students should be assured that they will be evaluated fairly on the published competencies of the course. The workload should be challenging but not overwhelming. Of course, there are many stressors in the lives of your students that you cannot control, but neither should you make the class more stressful than is inherent in the learning activity and its importance to the course objectives.

 PEARLS *Learning occurs best in psychologically and emotionally pleasant environments.*

Addressing Classroom Conduct

All behavior is motivated. Therefore, in addressing classroom conduct, it is essential to understand the motivation behind behavior, including classroom performance.

Student Motivation

motivation
An internal drive to achieve an unmet need.

Motivation occurs as a result of the student's experiencing dissatisfaction with the current state of affairs. That is, the learner must have an unmet need to be motivated. This unsatisfactory state of affairs can be either physical or psychological. It can be hunger, fear of physical harm, need for interaction with others, or a need to achieve personal satisfaction. Educationally, an individual is motivated to learn when his or her current state of knowledge is inadequate to perform as desired. Although instructors and others often speak about how to motivate students, the truth is that motivation is entirely internal. No person can give motivation to or cause motivation of another person. That having been said, as an instructor you can help students see how a particular activity or objective relates to his or her goals and can remove some barriers that divert an individual's actions away from his or her goals. There are two theories of motivation that will be helpful to you in deciding how to best approach the issue of student motivation.

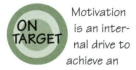 *Motivation is an internal drive to achieve an unmet need. Behavior is only motivated if its outcome is important to the individual.*

Expectancy Theory

expectancy theory
A theory that motivation results from the beliefs that efforts will lead to performance and that outcomes are related to performance when the outcome or reward is important to the individual.

Expectancy theory is based in three beliefs people have about their performance and goals (Greenburg and Baron 2000). These beliefs are expectancy, instrumentality, and valence. Expectancy refers to an individual's belief that his or her efforts will result in a desired performance. For example, students must have an expectancy, or expectation, that studying will lead to acceptable performance on an exam. Otherwise, they will not be motivated to study. Instrumentality refers to the belief that one's efforts will be rewarded according to his or her performance. That is, performance must be instrumental in being rewarded. There is little reason to perform if good performance and poor performance lead to the same outcomes. Finally, valance refers to the value a particular reward has for an individual. If the reward for performing well on a class project is being selected to receive free tuition to a seminar, the student will perform well only if going to the seminar is important to him or her. According to expectancy theory, effort must lead to performance, the reward for performance must be allocated according to the level or quality of performance, and the reward must be meaningful to the individual. It is not uncommon to hear students complain that it doesn't matter if they study or not, because the exam is not, or at least is perceived as not being, related to the objectives of the course.

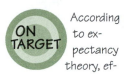 According to expectancy theory, effort must lead to performance, the reward for performance must be allocated according to the level or quality of performance, and the reward must be meaningful to the individual.

Maslow's Hierarchy of Needs

Maslow's hierarchy of needs
A theory that motivation occurs as needs are activated and met in order from more basic needs to higher-order needs.

Maslow's hierarchy of needs is a familiar conception of how individuals are motivated (Maslow 1943). Maslow's theory states that human behavior is aroused by unmet needs in a hierarchical manner, with lower-level, more-basic needs motivating behavior before higher-level needs are realized. Maslow's theory was never intended to be interpreted as a lockstep process. Simply, needs are activated generally in order from lowest to highest. The most basic needs are physiological, followed by safety needs, social needs, esteem needs, and self-actualization needs. Physiological needs include things such as food, water, and sleep. An individual cannot concentrate on other needs if deprived of food or other basic necessities of life. As an instructor, you can apply this information by allowing for adequate breaks in order for students to meet their physiological needs. Safety needs include both physical and psychological safety. This includes a physically safe learning environment and students feeling secure against psychological harm. Social needs refer to an individual's needs to be affiliated with and accepted by others. Social needs that are not met outside of class might be exposed in class in the form of excessive talkativeness. Allowing for adequate breaks can also help students meet their social needs for interaction with fellow students. Esteem needs include self-respect and recognition by others, including

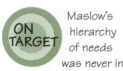

ON TARGET Maslow's hierarchy of needs was never intended to imply that higher-level needs could not be activated until lower-level needs are completely satisfied, but that lower-level needs must be satisfied to a sufficient degree before higher-level needs are activated.

achievement goal theory
A theory that students are motivated either by performance (demonstrating ability to others) or mastery (gaining proficiency).

classroom justice theory
A theory that motivation results from perceptions of fairness in terms of equity of performance and rewards as compared to the performance and rewards of others, specifically in the classroom setting.

instructors, for efforts and accomplishments. Finally, self-actualization needs refer to an individual's need to develop to his or her fullest potential. As an instructor, you can appeal to this need by showing how course content and activities will help the student perform at a high level.

Achievement Goal Theory and Classroom Justice Theory

There are other theories of motivation in addition to the ones just discussed. Some of these have been studied specifically in relation to student classroom performance. Two of these are **achievement goal theory** and **classroom justice theory.**

Students may be focused on either performance or mastery (Archer and Schevak 1998). The student with a performance orientation is concerned with demonstrating ability to others, or at least hiding lack of ability from others. Students with this orientation avoid challenging tasks if they doubt their ability to perform adequately. In order to appear competent, these students rely on superficial learning strategies, such as rote memorization. Mastery-oriented students are focused on becoming proficient and focus on effort rather than ability. Their desire is to understand material and processes. Therefore, they tend to use more-effective learning strategies for deeper processing and select more-challenging tasks.

Students perceive that teachers emphasize or reward one of these goal orientations over the other. Because having a mastery orientation is related to increased persistence in learning and a greater degree of learning, it is important to reward mastery. This can be done by assigning meaningful and interesting tasks of appropriate difficulty, giving feedback on strengths and weaknesses rather than just giving a score or grade, and giving students choices of tasks and choices in whether or not they will work collaboratively or individually on tasks. Mastery is not promoted when there is a competitive atmosphere in the classroom.

Most individuals in Western society are concerned with justice. Classroom justice is related to the **equity theory** of motivation (Chory-Assad 2002). According to equity theory, people compare their inputs and outputs in a situation to those of others with the expectation that these relationships will be equitable, or fair. Equity theory includes both distributive justice and procedural justice. Distributive justice refers to how resources and rewards are allocated—in other words, who gets what. **Procedural justice** refers to how decisions are made about who gets what. Students need to perceive that the policies and processes for grading, for example, are fair. Student perceptions of procedural justice increase performance motivation, enhance learning, and decrease student aggression toward instructors.

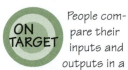

Student Conduct Issues

Although you will distribute your course policies and collect a signature of receipt for them at the beginning of your course, you will need to reintroduce expectations for conduct at times during the course. This can include establishing ground rules for participation in group activities or reminding participants that breaks are for a given number of minutes and class will begin again promptly at that time. Of course, you yourself must be ready to begin at the end of break, as well.

PEARLS Your conduct conveys to students what is acceptable. Students won't come back from break on time or refrain from using cell phones and pagers unless you do.

equity theory
A theory that motivation results from perceptions of fairness in terms of equity of performance and rewards as compared to the performance and rewards of others.

The purpose of your guidelines is to ensure a positive and productive learning atmosphere for all. Any behavior that disrupts this environment must be addressed. Many of these behaviors, such as punctuality, attendance, use of pagers and cellular phones, etc., can be addressed by course policy. With some regularity, however, you will need to address an issue on the spot in a way that puts an end to the dysfunctional behavior without further disrupting the learning environment. Dysfunctional behaviors often are not intended as such by the student and are therefore usually not disciplinary issues. There are a variety of reasons why students may not be doing what you expect them to (Mager and Pipe 1997). Your understanding of human motivation will provide insight into some of the behaviors described below and will assist you in addressing the behaviors. In general, there are some prototypical responses to common situations that you can adapt to the situation at hand.

PEARLS Before you address student behavior, attempt to understand its motivation. You will be more likely to address the behavior productively.

procedural justice
The perceived fairness of processes and policies related to the allocation of rewards.

Wilbert McKeachie (1994) has some excellent suggestions for handling a number of problem situations or "problem students." One of the most disconcerting of these situations is the hostile or aggressive student. Anger is often motivated by **goal interference** or perceptions of injustice and, not surprisingly, arises in response to the receipt of a less-than-expected grade. Anger may also arise during discussions that challenge a student's previously unquestioned point of view on a particular

goal interference
The perception that a particular situation, event, or individual is obstructing a person from achieving his or her objectives.

topic. Other issues include excessively talkative students, argumentative or know-it-all students, rigid students, complainers, dependent students, attention seekers, nonparticipation, and dishonesty (Donaldson and Scannell 1986; McClincy 1995; Parvensky 1995; McKeachie 1994). The following suggestions are just that—suggestions. They do not comprise an exhaustive list of how situations can be handled, nor are they intended to be a script; but they are meant to give you ideas about some ways of handling situations. In addition to specific suggestions, remember that affective grading can be used to address behaviors identified as incongruent with expected professional characteristics.

The Hostile, Confrontational Student

A sudden attack by a student can catch us off guard and make us defensive. This response can escalate the problem and, in any case, does nothing to resolve it. More than anything, the angry student wants to be heard. Therefore, the best thing you can do is to listen. Make it clear that you respect the student's point of view (even if you don't agree with it) by saying something like, "I can see how it might look that way from your point of view," or "I can see you have some concerns about this; tell me more about what you're thinking." From that point, you have some options. Is the issue over something factual or is it a matter of judgment? If, for example, a student is arguing about a response on an exam, you might ask him or her to bring you the source of information. If the student has information from a legitimate source, you may reconsider the student's original response to the question. You might pose the issue to the rest of the class and ask for other thoughts about the issue. Always consider that you may be wrong or at least incompletely correct. If this is the case, let the class or the individual student know that you will take the issue under consideration and provide a resolution at the next class. You must follow through with this. If the student has a valid point and you acknowledge it, students will gain respect for you. Avoid pressure to change a grade just to end the conflict. This is a slippery slope, and you will soon find students wanting consideration for clearly incorrect answers.

Talkative Students

Some students talk excessively in the course of class discussion, may have ongoing "sidebar" conversations, or may monopolize your time during breaks or office hours. Sometimes the talkative student is talking to a classmate about an idea from class and sometimes is talking about something irrelevant. Until you get to know students, you won't know into which category the student falls. Initially give the student the benefit of the doubt by asking if the student (or students) has something to contribute or if there is a question. If you come to find that the student talks to classmates and has nothing to contribute to the discussion, it may become necessary to call the student by name and say, for example, "Larry, can I have your attention please? This is information we all need to hear." Repeated offenses should lead to counseling the student outside of class. You should explain that your role is to make sure the entire class learns and that his or her talkativeness is interfering with that process.

For the student who monopolizes your time, make sure you give him or her fair consideration, but make it clear that you need to do something else. You could say, "Shanna, can you make an appointment to see me during office hours? We can discuss this then. I really need to take care of couple of things on break." Fortunately, most adults have well-developed social skills and recognize the cues we normally use to communicate. The talkative student often doesn't recognize these cues, so you need to be more explicit. When the student makes an appointment, make it clear how much time you have to spend. For example, say, "Dave, it's good to see you. We have 20 minutes right now, so tell me what's on your mind."

The know-it-all student can be a class time monopolizer. He or she may or may not be correct and is, in fact, a bit more challenging to handle when correct than when incorrect. One suggested response is, "Thanks, Bill. Let's hear what some of the others' ideas are." Remember, you don't have to call on the student every time he or she raises a hand, and you can use a direct question aimed at another student to circumvent the know-it-all's intent to answer so frequently. You can also ask particularly difficult questions of such students or ask them to explain their answers. This is particularly effective for the know-it-all who doesn't know so much, after all. Again, the know-it-all may be oblivious to social cues, and you may need to have a discussion with him or her outside of class. In doing so, make sure you acknowledge his or her contributions, but add that it is your job to hear from all the students.

 PEARLS Whenever possible, emphasize that your role is to act on behalf of the group. You'll be less likely to be perceived as having a personal issue with the student.

The Rigid Student

As you learned previously, past experiences can either be a help or a hindrance to subsequent learning. Past learning that has been deeply ingrained through drills or that has been reinforced by a lack of feedback on the appropriateness of performance can be a problem. The rigid student sees only one way of—or least a very limited number of options for—doing things. This can take the form of complaining about working in small groups because "the teacher is supposed to teach," arguing about skills being performed differently than the student was taught (i.e., "incorrectly"), or lack of success in laboratory and clinical scenarios because of the inability to adapt. Some suggestions for approaching this individual include asking the student to provide a rationale for his or her method or approach and posing scenarios in which the "usual way" won't work.

Complaining and Excuse-making Students

Occasionally you will have students who whine about just about everything, from "Why do we have to have a quiz today? That's not fair" to "Why don't you use the same kind of backboard straps in class that we use in our rescue squad?" Whiners can also be excuse makers and try to "negotiate" course standards and policies. The first thing to consider when confronted by a chronic complainer is whether or not the complaint might have merit. If the complaint relates to something that cannot be changed, such as class starting time or meeting days, let the student know that this is not something that can be changed. If the complaint has legitimacy, ask the student how he or she suggests it be handled. Deciding whether or not to accept a student's excuse for say, a late assignment, can be a dilemma. College students make deceptive excuses as frequently as legitimate excuses (McKeachie 1994). It is best to have clear policies regarding absences and late assignments. Because students do have legitimate extenuating circumstances at times, you should maintain the flexibility to be fair to these students. You may wish to tell students that, because of unforeseen circumstances, everyone gets one excused absence or late assignment, but that beyond that, you will need verifying documentation to consider being flexible.

Dependent Students

Sometimes you have students who come to you for guidance on every small matter and who seem to need an inordinate amount of direction. This can sometimes be due to anxiety and fear of failure. It is sometimes helpful to give a short, straightforward assignment or quiz or perhaps a "sample" assignment or quiz very early in the course so that students become aware of your expectations without risking academic success. Select this student to answer easy questions during class. This, too, will help the student build confidence. It is important to be supportive of students, but direct them toward independence.

Nonparticipating Students

There are a few reasons why students may not be participative in class. Anxiety and fear of being wrong can be handled much as for dependent students. Sometimes a student is shy, is insecure, or lacks confidence. Often, making eye contact with the student during class and smiling at him or her are reassuring. In this case, having students pair up with different partners or groups for class activities allows the student to become comfortable with classmates a little at a time and eventually to feel more comfortable interacting with the class as a whole. Sometimes the issue is that the student has not prepared for class. Attaching points to class participation can give the student an incentive to prepare and participate. Other students may be bored or may really lack understanding of the material and feel unable to participate. These students should be counseled on an individual basis.

Summary

In addition to effectively presenting content and skills in the classroom, as an instructor you are also responsible for managing the learning environment. This requires knowledge of what motivates behavior, what the characteristics of an effective learning environment are, and having a repertoire of prototypical responses to problem situations that you can adapt to the situation at hand. An effective classroom environment removes barriers to motivation and enhances student participation in the learning process. It is important that students are physically comfortable, are psychologically secure in the learning atmosphere, and have their needs for socialization and esteem respected. In addition, students learn more effectively if motivated for mastery rather than performance, if their expectations of justice are met, and if they believe their efforts will lead to being meaningfully rewarded.

REVIEW QUESTIONS

1. Explain the relationship between individual and group rights concerning classroom management.

2. List desirable physical characteristics of the classroom environment.

3. List desirable emotional characteristics of the classroom environment.

4. Discuss the relationship between motivation and behavior.

5. Describe the expectancy theory of motivation.

6. Describe the classroom justice theory of motivation.

7. Explain how you might manage a student who complains excessively and makes excuses.

Considerations in Laboratory and Clinical Teaching

Learning Objectives

Upon completion of this chapter you should be able to

- Discuss considerations for the effective administration of laboratory and clinical activities.

- Employ effective methods for teaching skills.

- Describe considerations in developing scenarios for laboratory practice.

- Discuss the purposes of clinical education.

- Describe the tasks of the clinical coordinator.

- Explain the need for clinical preceptor and lab instructor training.

- Discuss characteristics of effective clinical and laboratory learning situations.

- Explain the value of authenticity and fidelity in laboratory learning.

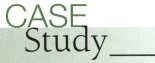

CASE Study_____

Dave Jennings has just been hired by Trendcare Ambulance Service as the clinical coordinator for BLS and ALS training programs. Dave will be responsible for making sure students are eligible for participating in clinical activities and scheduling students for their clinical rotations. Dave has worked as an instructor and preceptor before, but he has not performed the role of clinical coordinator.

Questions

1. What kinds of records do you think Dave will need to keep?
2. How will Dave know what the clinical sites expect of the program and the students?
3. What factors will Dave need to consider in scheduling students for clinical rotations?
4. What should Dave expect of the program preceptors?

Introduction

Achieving competence in professional practice requires effective learning opportunities in laboratory and clinical settings as well as classroom learning activities. Participation in lab and clinical settings functions not only to introduce additional knowledge, skills, and attitudes, but also to help students assimilate isolated pieces of knowledge and skill into integrated practice. Meaningful lab and clinical experiences don't just happen but must be thoughtfully constructed. The purpose of this chapter is to provide you with some principles and ideas for successful laboratory and clinical teaching.

KEY TERMS

authenticity, p. 296	clinical coordinator, p. 291	internship, p. 289
clinical affiliation agreement, p. 292	clinical education, p. 288	preceptor, p. 290
	fidelity, p. 296	proficiency, p. 289

Clinical Education

clinical education
The portion of an educational program that takes place in the service setting.

Clinical education deserves specific attention because it is often the least well-developed portion of educational programs. It is important to appreciate what clinical education is and what its purposes are in order to understand the importance of preceptor training and the deliberate arrangement of clinical experiences. We do not differentiate here between field clinical and hospital clinical settings. The term *internship*, or *field internship*, is sometimes inappropriately used to refer to all learning

internship
The final phase of clinical education, which takes place in the field setting for the purpose of the student demonstrating competency.

activities that take place in the prehospital setting. In EMS, the **internship** is the final portion of clinical education that takes place in the prehospital, or field, setting for the purpose of allowing students to demonstrate entry-level competence as they continue to refine their practice.

Definitions of Clinical Education

The following definitions provide insight into the importance of clinical education. According to Moore and Perry (1976, 421) clinical education is

> . . . that portion of a student's professional education that involves practice and application of classroom knowledge and skills to on the job responsibilities. It is a participative experience with limited time spent in observation.

Mary Lee Seibert (1979, 368) provides a complementary definition of clinical education:

> That part of the education process in a health profession that takes place in the service setting and has the purpose of allowing students to practice, under competent supervision, the knowledge, skills, and attitudes learned in the classroom and lab.

PEARLS We learn by doing—students must be able to participate in the clinical setting in order to learn effectively.

Purposes of Clinical Education

proficiency
A level of skill performance that includes both competency and efficiency.

In the clinical setting students have the opportunity to develop **proficiency** as health-care providers. Proficiency is the combination of skill and speed, or efficiency and effectiveness. Practice becomes both competent and efficient. Students are exposed to the work environment, which provides a context for the application of knowledge and skills and allows them to observe role models and begin being socialized into the occupation. Guided participation in clinical activities allows students to develop problem-solving and critical-thinking skills—that is, to think like an EMS provider (Schön 1987). Clinical activities should be directed toward the student's development of independence, work-organization skills, decision-making skills, and assumption of responsibility.

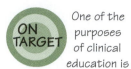

One of the purposes of clinical education is to help students learn to think like EMS providers.

Students must not be allowed just to practice skills in the clinical setting, but must be allowed to recognize and solve problems as they will be expected to do as providers.

The essence of clinical education is that the student must develop a repertoire of experience with actual situations that can later be drawn upon to solve previously unencountered problems. This requires reflection on experiences. However, students often lack the frame of reference through which to reflect upon experiences. It is incumbent on the preceptor to ask the appropriate questions to push the student through the experiential learning cycle (see Chapter 7) (Harrelson and Leaver-Dunn, 2002). This process enables the student to build and refine schemas, which can then serve to enable recognition of problems and as rules for formulating solutions for them.

The ability to recognize and solve problems is critical for transitioning to the world of work, because work consists of a series of problems to be solved. Thus, problem-solving is the key to getting work done. The preceptor assists the student by having the student verbalize his recognition of the problem—that is, what *is* versus what *should be* in the situation. The student must then be able to define the desired outcomes of the situation and devise and implement a plan to achieve the outcomes.

Preceptors

preceptor
A competent provider who is willing and able to teach students in the clinical setting.

A **preceptor** is a teacher who is a competent clinical practitioner willing and able to take responsibility for teaching and evaluating students in the work setting. Preceptors function as professional role models after which students can pattern their behavior. Box 19-1 lists the characteristics of effective preceptors, and Box 19-2 lists the tasks expected of preceptors. In order for preceptors to effectively carry out these tasks

Box 19-1

Characteristics of Effective Preceptors

- Effective communicator
- Interested in students
- Enthusiastic
- Organized
- Knows how to teach
- Clinically competent
- Provides honest but tactful feedback
- Open-minded
- Respectful

Box19-2

Tasks and Expectations of the Preceptor

- Welcomes students into the work setting.
- Orients students to the work setting.
- Introduces students to others.
- Provides information to students.
- Interacts with students.
- Reviews expectations with students.
- Assesses students' learning.
- Creates opportunities for learning.
- Allows student to participate.
- Guides student performance.
- Stimulates critical, reflective thinking.
- Gives feedback.
- Communicates with the educational program.

and responsibilities, it is essential that they attend a clinical education workshop that addresses practices in clinical education as well as specific program information and expectations.

PEARLS Preceptors are not just competent clinical providers but are instructors, as well. As such, they must have the opportunity to develop instructional skills.

Administration of Clinical Education

Clinical Coordination

clinical coordinator
The individual responsible for the administration of the clinical portion of the educational program.

Clinical coordination is largely an administrative matter. The **clinical coordinator's** job is facilitated by the existence of clear, comprehensive clinical education policies and a student clinical handbook. Two key responsibilities of the clinical coordinator are scheduling and documenting student achievement.

Scheduling can be accomplished in a number of ways, either on paper or electronically. In either instance, it is essential to know on what days students may attend particular sites or units, what shifts are available, and how many students can be accommodated per shift. It is a good, and often required, practice to establish a deadline for clinical scheduling in order to allow sufficient time to communicate the schedule to clinical-site personnel. Depending on specific program policies, students may either be able to sign up for shifts made available on the schedule, or the clinical coordinator may assign a schedule to the students. In either case, it is important to schedule specific clinical rotations in relationship to classroom and lab activities by correlating the schedule with the course syllabus. FISDAP™, created by Headwaters Software, is a clinical scheduling and competency-tracking package created specifically for EMS education. Other scheduling programs, both generic and specific to clinical education, exist as well.

Each program has minimum requirements for the number of clinical hours spent in specific areas as well as minimum requirements for specific competencies. It is essential that there is a mechanism for verifying student-reported activities. Records must be kept up to date, and progress reports must be given to students on a regular basis. This can be done by using a commercial product for clinical tracking or by using an Excel™ spreadsheet.

The clinical coordinator may also be responsible for collecting documentation establishing students' eligibility for clinical rotations. This may include verification of health requirements, such as immunizations, requesting criminal history checks, keeping records of CPR training and EMT-Basic certification, student signatures acknowledging receipt of clinical policies, and copies of student waivers. Finally, the clinical coordinator acts as the liaison between the educational program and the clinical sites and typically serves as the contact person for both students and clinical sites.

Clinical Affiliation Agreements and Student Waivers

clinical affiliation agreement
A legal document specifying the rights and responsibilities of both the educational institution and the clinical site.

Clinical affiliation agreements are legal agreements between an educational program and its clinical sites specifying the conditions under which the clinical site will permit students to participate in patient care in their facility or agency. The agreement addresses liability and indemnity issues and may be specific as to scheduling, preceptor qualifications, and tasks students are permitted or not permitted to carry out. Most larger institutions and agencies already have a preferred format for the agreement. If you are amending an existing agreement or generating a new agreement, it is important to seek out the legal counsel for your organization. Clinical agreements may be valid for a variable amount of time, and expiration dates must be tracked so that agreements can be renewed without a lapse. In addition to the clinical agreement, many agencies and institutions require students to sign an individual waiver of liability, confidentiality agreement, or other document verifying understanding of institutional expectations and policies.

Laboratory Education

The purpose of the laboratory component of an educational program goes beyond teaching a collection of disconnected skills. The lab must also set the stage for the transfer of learning into the clinical environment and promote integration of discrete skills into fluid practice. There are special considerations for the techniques and educational environment for the teaching-learning interaction in the laboratory setting. To frame the discussion of these considerations, review the two classification systems for the levels within the psychomotor domain of learning in Boxes 19-3 and 19-4.

The Teaching-Learning Transaction in the Psychomotor Domain

Learning skills is a much more complex process than it may seem. Teaching skills brings us to the realization that, in the words of Michael Polanyi (1966), we know more than we can say. The knowledge involved in clinical practice, both in terms of problem recognition and skill performance, exists both implicitly and explicitly. Success in teaching problem recognition and skill performance depends partly upon the ability to make implicit knowledge explicit and communicate it to the learner. The process of task analysis is based upon making the implicit knowledge of a skill explicit. Yet there are some elements of problem recognition and skill performance that cannot be verbalized. This knowledge remains tacit and must be learned through experience. For example, we cannot adequately verbalize the tactile sensation of the way bag-valve-mask ventilations feel

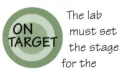

The lab must set the stage for the transfer of learning into the clinical environment and promote integration of discrete skills into fluid practice.

Box 19-3

Levels in the Psychomotor Domain, According to Dave
(Dave 1967)

Level	Description
Imitation	Copies the performance of an observed skill.
Manipulation	Performs a skill following general instructions rather than relying on observation.
Precision	Performs the skill independently and proficiently
Articulation	Can adapt the skill to fit new situations and can combine skills in series
Naturalization	The skill is automatic, performed with minimal effort

Box 19-4

Levels in the Psychomotor Domain, According to Simpson
(Simpson 1972)

Level	Description
Perception	Uses sensory cues to guide skill performance
Set	Awareness of the circumstances under which the skill is to be performed; readiness to act
Guided response	Analogous to Dave's imitation and manipulation
Mechanism	Performs skill correctly, not necessarily smoothly or efficiently
Complex overt response	Performs the skill smoothly, efficiently
Adaptation	Modifies the skill to adapt to new situations
Origination	Develops a "style" that replaces the skill as it was originally learned

when they are performed correctly, with a good seal, nor can we explain the feeling of increased lung resistance. Nonetheless, there is a critical role for the instructor in the laboratory setting.

Alexander Romiszowski (2004) lists five stages or phases of the student experience of acquiring skills (Box 19-5). The activities of the teaching-learning transaction in the lab must consider these stages. George and Doto's (2001) five-step method for teaching psychomotor

Box 19-5

Romiszowski's Stages of Skill Development
(Romiszowski 2004)

- Stage 1: Acquiring knowledge of what should be done, why it should be done, what the sequence is, and how the skill is carried out.
- Stage 2: Execution of the skill in a step-by-step manner.
- Stage 3: Transfer of control from the eyes to the kinesthetic control of muscles.
- Stage 4: Automation of skills.
- Stage 5: Generalization of skills.

Box 19-6

George and Doto's Five-Step Method of Teaching/Learning Clinical Skills
(George and Doto 2001)

- **Step 1: Conceptualization.** The student must understand the cognitive aspects of the skill, its indications, contraindications, tools used, and precautions to be taken.
- **Step 2: Visualization.** The student must see the entire skill performed in real time.
- **Step 3: Verbalization.** The student needs to hear a narrative of the procedure as each step is performed. The student should also be able to verbalize the steps.
- **Step 4: Practice.** This may include practice of skill subcomponents prior to practicing the skill as a whole.
- **Step 5: Correction and Reinforcement.** Errors must be corrected immediately to avoid having the student "learn" incorrectly through flawed practice.

skills (Box 19-6) reflects the phases described by Romiszowski. Their method is consistent with the concept of "whole-part-whole" learning discussed in previous chapters.

Learning skills is sometimes fraught with difficulty and frustration for students. A number of factors may account for deficits in student performance. These include strengths and weaknesses in learners' traits and abilities, inadequate or inappropriate description or demonstration of the skill, imprinting of incorrect or obsolete techniques through prior practice and experience, improper correction or reinforcement, and student affective issues.

The Importance of Fidelity in the Lab

ON TARGET *Learning is contextual. The more realistic the simulations and scenarios in a lab are, the greater the likelihood that learning will be transferred into the clinical setting.*

Learning is contextual. The more realistic the simulations and scenarios in the lab are, the greater the likelihood that learning will be transferred into the clinical setting. When laboratory practice is not *authentic,* students end up learning two parallel ways of doing things: one for the lab and one for "real life." Unfortunately, EMS instructors are faced with the seemingly dichotomous practices of preparing students for a stereotypical practical examination and preparing students for the complexities and unpredictability of real-life practice. Skill evaluation checklists should be seen as basic principles of skills that can be accomplished in more than one way, rather than rigid prescriptions for skill performance.

It is important that students learn the principles of skills in such a manner that they become automated. Students must understand that maintaining the integrity of the principles of the skill is much more important than arguing about the use of one particular technique for achieving the principles over another. Once students learn the basic components of a skill, the skill should be practiced under a variety of circumstances to allow students the opportunity to see that a rigid, lockstep approach will leave them unable to accomplish the task in many situations.

fidelity
The degree to which something is true to its real-life counterpart.

Fidelity refers to the faithfulness of laboratory conditions to real life—that is, how authentic the laboratory conditions are. Too often, laboratory practice is not authentic. Students enter the scene with hands raised, chanting, "Scene safety, BSI," without being able even to say what they would look for in terms of safety at a particular scene or what type of BSI would be appropriate. Scenarios are constructed in which a chair and table serve as the driver's seat and dash of a motor vehicle, students are never made to take off their classmates' shoes and socks and actually locate a pedal or posterior tibial pulse, and students recite that they are "looking for DCAP-BTLS" without assessing the mock patient in a manner that would actually reveal any abnormalities. Students perform their assessments in a cursory manner, going through the motions without ever concentrating on the look, feel, and sound of "normal" so that they may recognize "not normal" when they encounter it. **Authenticity** is critical and must be a goal of all laboratory sessions.

authenticity
The degree to which something is representative of its real-life counterpart.

Constructing Lab Scenarios

Constructing quality lab scenarios requires time and a template for ensuring that all necessary information is provided to students. Real-life situations are a rich resource for scenario ideas. Regardless of whether scenarios are based on actual events or created from scratch, they should contain all the information a provider would expect to notice as he or she approaches and enters the scene. Other information, including assessment findings, patient history, and changes in the patient's condition, must be available to the lab instructor but should not be provided to the student unless he or she asks for it or performs the actions necessary to elicit the information. Care should be taken that vital signs, patient behavior, and other factors are consistent with the picture you are trying to paint for the student. Presenting your scenarios to another EMS provider before class will help you pinpoint inconsistencies and missing information. When constructing scenarios, you should take the time to prepare some questions for student group discussion.

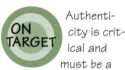

Authenticity is critical and must be a goal of all laboratory sessions.

PEARLS Using a template to construct lab scenarios helps ensure the appropriate information is included in each scenario.

Administrative Components of the Lab

You may find yourself in the role of lab coordinator as part of your instructional role. It is important that lab sessions be well planned and organized. The coordination functions related to lab sessions may include scheduling and briefing assistant instructors, setting up and breaking down lab rooms and equipment, and organizing student rotations.

The selection of lab instructors will vary with state and institutional policies. W. D. McClincy (1995) offers the following suggestions for selecting lab instructors.

- Lab instructors must be able to demonstrate proficiency in the skills he or she will be teaching and evaluating.
- Lab instructors should, at a minimum, be certified at the level of instruction they teach.
- Lab instructors must be positive role models.
- Lab instructors should be motivated by the desire to teach, rather than by recognition or financial compensation.
- Lab instructors must be reliable.
- Lab instructors must be knowledgeable in and demonstrate effective skill-teaching techniques.
- Lab instructors must be reputable and respected within their EMS service area.

In some states, only providers who have completed training offered or endorsed by the state EMS regulatory body may serve as skill instructors or evaluators. Whether or not this is the case, you should discuss your expectations with any lab instructors or evaluators you use. Lab instructors must agree to teach in a manner consistent with the way the program teaches students to perform skills, to use effective instructional and feedback techniques, and to fairly evaluate students based on the program's standards.

 PEARLS Some states require that EMS lab instructors and/or evaluators be endorsed by the state EMS regulatory body.

The number of lab instructors and the amount of space and equipment you will need depends upon the number of students you have and the purpose of the lab. Early on, an ideal student-to-instructor ratio is 4:1. When skills are first being introduced and practiced, students must be under constant supervision so that performance can be monitored and errors can be corrected immediately, before they become imprinted. Later, as students become more competent, they can monitor each other's performance with less direct supervision by lab instructors.

Summary

The laboratory and clinical components of an EMS program provide learning experiences that cannot be achieved in the classroom. There are special considerations in both settings for constructing effective teaching-learning opportunities. Clinical education depends heavily upon the quality of the interaction between the student and preceptor. The preceptor plays a critical role in helping the student engage in reflection on experience so that experiences are made meaningful and contribute positively to subsequent experience. In the lab, the use of effective instructional techniques by lab instructors and attention to the fidelity of simulations and authenticity of scenarios are key to student learning.

REVIEW QUESTIONS

1. Describe characteristics of effective clinical education experiences.

2. What are the purposes of clinical education?

3. Discuss the characteristics of effective clinical preceptors.

4. Describe how laboratory learning can best be transferred to clinical practice.

5. Discuss considerations in constructing effective laboratory scenarios.

6. Discuss characteristics of effective laboratory instructors.

CHAPTER 20

Roles and Responsibilities of Key Institutions and Personnel

Learning Objectives

Upon completion of this chapter you should be able to

- Discuss the general organizational structure related to EMS education in academic institutions, public safety agencies, and hospitals.

- Discuss the roles and responsibilities of program and institutional administrative personnel.

- List the types of agencies that might have oversight of EMS programs in your state.

- Discuss the roles and responsibilities of faculty.

- State the responsibilities and qualifications for the EMS educational program director and medical director.

- Discuss the roles of admissions departments and the office of the registrar in the higher education system.

- Model effective interactions with clerical and support staff.

- Differentiate between the meanings of role and title.

- Explain the purpose of faculty organizations.

CASE
Study____

A bby Collingsworth has been an EMS instructor in a hospital-based program for 10 years. She is delighted that she has been offered the faculty position she applied for in the EMS program at Byrd State University, but she is a little overwhelmed by all the unfamiliar titles and roles in the organizational chart. Abby's previous program was so small that she did most of her clerical work herself. Now she will have a support person to help her with some of these tasks. Working in an academic institution will certainly be a change!

Questions

1. How would you explain to Abby the roles of academic administrators, such as chancellors, provosts, deans, and presidents?
2. How would you describe to Abby the different designations of assistant, associate, adjunct, and clinical faculty members?
3. What advice would you give Abby about interacting with program support personnel?

Introduction

W hether you are new to teaching or have been doing it for some time, the organizational structure and administrative roles and functions of individuals in educational institutions or departments can seem like a morass. In order to function most effectively, it is important that you understand the general roles and responsibilities of key individuals in your institution and that you are aware of the external regulatory bodies that may have oversight of your program. The purpose of this chapter is to provide a general overview of organizational structure in various settings in which EMS education may occur and to summarize the roles and responsibilities associated with key personnel.

Organizational Structures

Academic Institutions

In both community colleges and universities there is a general common organizational structure. In some institutions, EMS is a department within a school in the college or university, and in others it is a program within another department such as nursing or health sciences. Some institutions operate under a chancellor, and others operate under a president. The hierarchy under the president may include a provost and/or a chancellor. Vice presidents may operate directly under the president or under the chancellor. Deans and directors (e.g., director of libraries, etc.) may answer to the provost, chancellor, or a vice president. Each of these positions may be qualified with terms such as assistant, associate, senior associate, or executive. Deans operate more narrowly in the system, with responsibilities in a particular school or university service, such as student affairs. Department or program chairs are organized under a dean. Program directors function under a department chair. Faculty function under a department chair or program director and may include instructors, assistant professors, associate professors, and professors. Faculty members may be full-time, part-time, adjunct, or affiliate. Adjunct or affiliate appointments do not constitute a regular employment relationship with the institution. In medicine and the health sciences, the additional qualifier of *clinical*—i.e., clinical assistant professor—designates a role only in the clinical setting. Although there may be some variations, typically the organizational structure is similar to that in Figure 20-1.

In addition to the faculty, administrative support personnel, such as financial managers, secretaries, student advisors, and executive assistants, are vital to the smooth operation of an academic program.

Qualifications, Roles, and Responsibilities of Program Personnel

In order to obtain and maintain accreditation by the Committee on Accreditation of Education Programs for the Emergency Medical Services Professions (CoAEMSP), programs must adhere to the guidelines established by the CoAEMSP (1999). Keep in mind that job titles are determined by the employer and may not directly coincide with the roles described here. That is, someone with a job title of EMS Education Coordinator may function in the capacity of program director for the purposes of accreditation.

Program Direction

Program leadership and management responsibilities may be carried out by one or more individuals who must be qualified to perform the duties stated in the job description. The program director is ultimately responsible for all aspects of the program, including

- Administration, organization, and supervision of the educational program.
- Continuous quality improvement for the program.

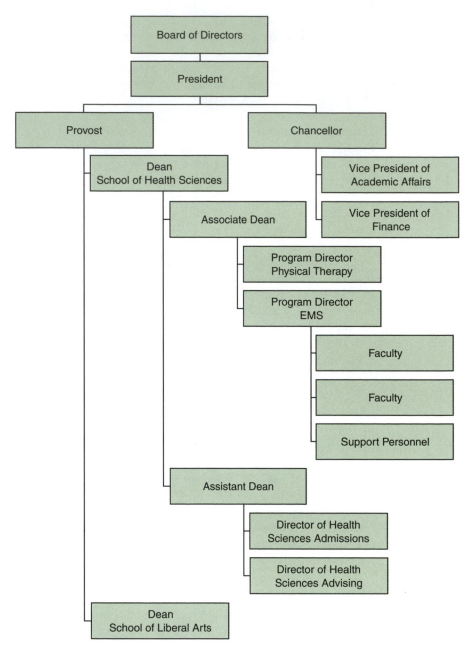

Figure 20-1
Academic Institution Organizational Chart

- Long-range planning and continued development of the program.
- Program effectiveness.
- Cooperative involvement with the program medical director.
- Delegation of responsibilities.

The program director must possess a minimum of a bachelor's degree from an accredited institution of higher education and, in many cases, must hold a master's degree in order to perform the responsibilities of the position. The CoAEMSP standards further require that the program director has "appropriate education, training, and experience to fulfill the responsibilities of this position" and must be "knowledgeable about methods on [sic] instruction, testing, and evaluation of students." The program director must have field experience and should be certified as a paramedic by a nationally recognized certifying organization. The program director must also be knowledgeable about national curricula, national accreditation, national registration, and the requirements for state certification (CoAEMSP 1994).

 PEARLS The emphasis is on program direction, rather than program director, indicating that these responsibilities may be shared.

Medical Direction

The medical director is responsible for the medical aspects of a program and is accountable for the following:

- Reviewing and approving educational content for appropriateness and accuracy.
- Reviewing and approving the quality of medical instruction and student evaluation.
- Reviewing and approving the progress of each student throughout the program.
- Attesting to the competence of all graduates in all domains of learning.
- Cooperative involvement with the program director.
- Delegation of responsibilities as appropriate.

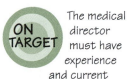 **ON TARGET** The medical director must have experience and current knowledge of emergency medicine and must also have knowledge or experience in prehospital care and be knowledgeable about EMS education.

The medical director must be a licensed physician in the United States and have experience and current knowledge of emergency medicine. He or she must also have training and/or experience in the delivery of prehospital care, must be an active member of the local medical community, and must be knowledgeable about paramedic education (CoAEMSP 1999).

Faculty

The instructional faculty are responsible for coordination and delivery of instruction and assessment of student achievement. Faculty must be knowledgeable in course content and must use effective instructional methods. The full-time lead instructor should be certified by a nationally recognized certification body. In addition to the faculty, the program must have adequate support staff (CoAEMSP 1999).

In addition to the CoAEMSP standards, there may be other faculty responsibilities, depending on the institution for which you work. These responsibilities can include serving on school, college, or university committees, scholarship (research and publication), and professional service, such as participating in professional organizations, consulting, or volunteering.

Faculty Organizations

Most institutions have some form of faculty governance, such as a faculty senate, that can pass resolutions concerning faculty affairs. Some institutions have faculty bargaining units to represent faculty rights to the institutional administration. Some issues that may be handled by a collective bargaining unit include compensation, workload, promotion, academic freedom, and similar issues. The faculty senate functions in a broad manner to inquire into and pass resolutions concerned with the academic function of the university. A faculty senate may have several committees to monitor specific issues.

College and University Administrative Units

As a faculty member, you will need some familiarity with the functions of various departments in your institution, because students often approach faculty with questions that should be referred to the appropriate office. Typically, you must have information about the admissions' department, registrar's office, and bursar's office. Your institution may have both an institutional and a school or program admissions' officer. The function of admissions is to process student applications and determine if students have met the prerequisites for entry into the program. Students should be directed to the registrar for any difficulties in registering for classes or receiving official course grades. The bursar's office deals with tuition bills, disbursement of financial aid, and payment. In some institutions these functions may be handled by a finance or billing office.

Public Safety Institutions and Ambulance Services

Many fire departments and ambulance services have training academies or education departments. In fire departments the training-academy administrator may be a career officer or a civilian employee.

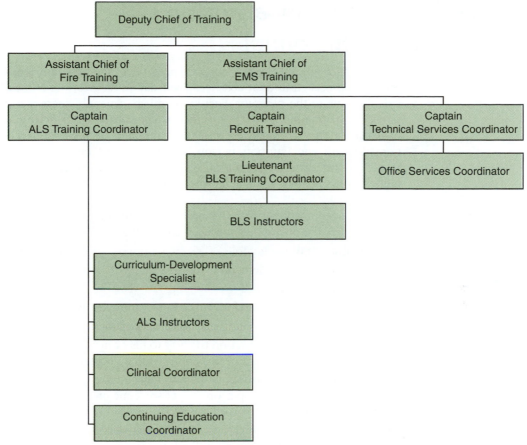

Figure 20-2
Fire Department Training Academy Organizational Chart

One typical structure is represented in Figure 20-2. Ambulance services that do not operate similarly to fire departments may have a training officer or, if larger, an education department. EMS education programs are sometimes under common administration with CQI programs.

Hospital-based Programs

Hospital-based EMS education programs may be part of a hospital-based ambulance service or may function as part of the hospital education department or the emergency department. It is in this situation that a variety of organizational structures is most likely to occur.

A Special Note on Interacting with Support Personnel

Clerical and administrative support personnel are generally most acutely appreciated in their absence. Their day-to-day work is of incalculable value to the program. Faculty members generally share a support person and often give work to that person without considering his or her additional workload. In order to maintain a good working relationship with your support person, he or she must be treated with respect as an individual and with respect for his or her overall responsibilities. Some pointers to facilitate this relationship are as follows:

- Take a genuine interest in this person as a human being. Don't talk to him or her only when you want something.
- Say please and thank you.
- Ask. Don't order or demand.
- Don't micromanage.
- Give sufficient lead time for him or her to complete your task.
- Encourage dialogue about workload and deadlines.
- Don't walk past the copier on the way to his or her desk just to ask him or her to make four or five copies—do it yourself.
- If a phone call is important enough to make, make it yourself. Don't ask your support person to "get someone on the line" for you. It is rude to both parties involved.
- Show appreciation. Don't forget administrative assistants' day. Buy a cup of coffee for or give a small gift to your support person when he or she really goes out of his or her way to help you out of a bind.

 PEARLS *Good administrative support personnel are the glue that holds the program together.*

Outside Agencies

Your program may be required to follow guidelines set forth by a variety of agencies or regulatory bodies, depending upon the type and location of your program. You may need to be aware of guidelines and standards required by your state's commission or department of education or higher education as well as those of your state's EMS regulatory body. Your institution may be accredited by bodies other than the CoAEMSP, such as the North Central Association on Accreditation or the Council for Higher Education Accreditation.

Summary

No matter where you teach or in what type of institution, an understanding of the administrative structure and function of the organization will make things a bit less confusing. Knowing your roles and responsibilities and those of other key program personnel and departments make for smoother program operation. One of the key but often overlooked roles in educational programs is that of administrative support. Your relationship with your support person is one worth investing in. Finally, it is important to be aware that educational programs often have to meet the standards of a variety of outside organizations in addition to those of the CoAEMSP for accredited programs and those of your state's EMS regulatory body.

REVIEW QUESTIONS

1. Describe the responsibilities of the program director.

2. Describe the responsibilities of the medical director.

3. Describe the responsibilities of the faculty.

4. Discuss ways to establish and maintain a good working relationship with administrative support personnel.

Career
and Professional
Development

Learning Objectives

Upon completion of this chapter you should be able to

- Describe the importance of continuing professional development.

- Discuss the importance of belonging to professional organizations.

- Explain the value of attending professional conferences.

- Explore avenues for undergraduate and/or graduate education.

- Discuss the benefits of writing for publication.

- Suggest avenues for professional networking.

- List venues where EMS education jobs are commonly posted.

- Distinguish between the formats of résumés and curricula vitae.

- Discuss the use of professional portfolios.

- Plan for a job interview.

- List considerations in deciding whether or not to accept a job offer.

- Value the importance of research, writing, and presenting in professional development.

CASE
Study____

E d English has worked as an adjunct instructor for Belmont University's EMS program for 4 years. Now that he is eligible for retirement from his fire-department position, he is looking for a full-time job in EMS education. A native of Mississippi, Ed is thinking that somewhere where there is a lot of snow in the wintertime might give him the chance to ski and snowmobile, two activities he hasn't had much of an opportunity to do.

Questions

1. Where would you advise Ed to begin his job search?
2. What advice would you give Ed concerning his CV or résumé?
3. What questions would you encourage Ed to ask during his interviews?

Introduction

Y ou've reached the point where you're ready to put your new knowledge and skills to use. In preparation for doing so, it is important to remember that this is only the beginning of your professional development. Regardless of your intended level of involvement in education— whether you will occasionally teach in an adjunct capacity or whether you aspire to be full-time instructional staff or faculty or even a program director—it is critical that you participate in professional development activities. The purpose of this chapter is to provide an overview of professional development and to give some practical information about job searches.

KEY TERMS

curriculum vita, curricula vitae (pl.), p. 313

lifelong learning, p. 311

malapropisms, p. 313

networking, p. 311

portfolio, p. 313

professional journal, p. 313

realistic job preview, p. 317

résumé, p. 313

trade magazine, p. 313

Continuing Professional Development

lifelong learning
A never-ending quest for personal and professional growth.

Education is a vast field philosophically, theoretically, and practically. Not only should you review information from time to time in order to reconsider it in light of your increasing experience, you will never run out of new things to learn about education. We all succumb to day-to-day pressures and fall into a comfortable routine in our teaching because it saves us time. In order to meet the challenge of **lifelong learning** and growth, we all need to take time to evaluate our teaching practices and add to our repertoire of methods. We also need to maintain current knowledge of our content areas. Knowledge and practices in medicine and health sciences change rapidly. If you truly have a love for teaching and for your content areas, this will not seem burdensome, though admittedly, finding the time and resources can be a little challenging.

 PEARLS *Lifelong learning is critical for both personal and professional development.*

networking
Meeting and interacting with professional mentors and peers to exchange ideas and learn about opportunities.

There are a variety of venues for continuing professional development. Many university schools of education and departments of faculty development have excellent Web sites. Professional organizations generally hold annual conferences that are not only an excellent source for professional development, but also a way of meeting and **networking** with colleagues. The National Association of EMS Educators (NAEMSE) meets annually in September and offers a variety of tracks, topics, and speakers. Other EMS conferences, such as EMS Today, sponsored by *JEMS*, and EMS Expo, sponsored by the National Association of EMTs, offer both content sessions and education tracks.

Professional Organizations

Belonging to professional organizations offers a number of benefits. Membership generally entails a reduced fee for conferences, belonging to listservs, the ability to serve on committees, and subscription to newsletters or other publications. In some cases, your employer will pay your annual membership dues.

Attending your organizations' conferences allows you to meet people who are active at state, national, and even international levels in EMS education. You have the opportunity to meet program directors and faculty from other programs. Networking with these individuals can lead to recommendations for committee service and task forces, employment opportunities, and other professional opportunities. Talking with other instructors allows you to exchange ideas and gain different perspectives on educational practices and issues. To maximize the benefits of networking, always keep a supply of your business cards with you.

Organizational membership affords you the opportunity to stay up to date with trends and issues in EMS and EMS education via newsletters and listservs. Organizational newsletters may also allow you opportunities to write for publication. Being active on committees of professional organizations allows you to make a difference in EMS education through position papers and projects.

Formal Education

You may wish at some point to increase your expertise in the field of education by pursuing a bachelor's degree or, if you already have an undergraduate degree, a master's or doctoral degree. If you are teaching in an institution of higher education, you will generally be required to have a degree that is one level of education beyond that offered by the program in which you are teaching. Increasingly, your opportunities in the private sector and in public safety are limited without at least a bachelor's degree.

You may wish to pursue a general degree in adult education or a more specialized degree in health sciences education, curriculum and instruction, educational administration, instructional design systems, or instructional technology. As you become more involved in education, you will find areas that especially appeal to you.

Whether you take classes part-time or full-time or on-campus or via distance education, you must ensure that you are taking classes from an accredited college or university. This is necessary not only if you are applying for financial aid, but also to afford you credibility in your field. Reputable employers will not hire you for degree-required positions unless your degree is from an accredited educational institution. As with most things, if it sounds too good to be true, it probably is. Quality education takes time. Programs offering nearly instantaneous degrees generally do not provide you with a quality education.

PEARLS Make sure any colleges or universities you attend are accredited by recognized regional higher-education accreditation bodies.

Job Seeking

Résumés, Curricula Vitae, and Portfolios

Whether or not you are actively seeking a position, you should always have an up-to-date **résumé** or **curriculum vita** available. In academia, you will be required to submit a curriculum vita (CV) to be considered for employment, and in most other situations, you will submit a résumé. Because a résumé is briefer, you may want to supplement it with a **portfolio** of your work.

The essential difference between a résumé and a curriculum vita is that a résumé hits the highlights of your education and employment and should be no longer than one page, whereas a CV is comprehensive and contains detailed descriptions of your academic preparation and work experience, as well as publications, presentations, and other information. For either document, it is absolutely critical that spelling, grammar, syntax, punctuation, and format be faultless. Misspellings, poor grammar, and **malapropisms,** or misuse of words, are poor reflections on someone who will be in a position to teach others. (*Author's note*: In one memorable instance, some colleagues and I reviewed a CV in which the applicant stated he had graduated "cum latte" rather than cum laude [with honors].) Figures 21-1 and 21-2 show examples of the format for résumés and CVs. Finally, your résumé or CV should be on quality résumé paper, which can be obtained at business stationery stores or office supply stores.

A portfolio is a collection of exemplars of your work. Depending on the type of job you are seeking, it may contain lesson plans, presentations, examples of forms or documents you have created, or other work relevant to the position.

Job Searches

EMS education jobs are not typically advertised in general media, such as newspapers or general job-search Web sites. The best ways of finding out about jobs in EMS education are through professional publications and Web sites and by word of mouth (an important reason for networking). EMS education jobs may be found in professional organization newsletters, state EMS newsletters, and **trade magazines,** such as *JEMS, Emergency Medical Services,* and *Firehouse.* Many trade magazines have online versions, as well. **Professional journals** such as *Prehospital Emergency Care* and *Academic Emergency Medicine* also list employment opportunities. Many EMS-related websites, such as those of the National

Figure 21-1
Résumé Format

Phyllis Smith
2021 Pinewood Ct.
Johnsonville, WA 99999
(899) 555-1111
psmith@rcom.com

Employment History

1999–Present	Fernwood Fire Department, Fernwood, WA. Started as an EMT-B/firefighter I at the rank of private. Promoted to lieutenant in 2002 after completing EMT-P training. Primary responsibility was responding to EMS and fire calls. Transferred to the training academy in 2003. Primary responsibilities are skills teaching in recruit classes and continuing education programs, and occasional lecturing.
1994–1999	Johnson County Ambulance Service, Johnsonville, WA. EMT-B. Responsible for BLS patient care and assisting with ALS patient care.

Volunteer Experience

1995–Present	EMT-B with Reynolds Rescue Squad. Responsible for responding on emergency medical calls in a rural setting.

Education

1991–1995	Attended Epiphany College. Graduated with honors with a bachelor of arts degree in European literature. Member of Phi Omega sorority and Golden Key honor society. GPA: 3.6/4.0.
2003	Completed EMS Primary Instructor training at Middlefork Community College, Middlefork, WA.
2001–2002	Completed EMT-P certificate program at the Fernwood, WA, Fire Department Training Academy.
1994	Completed EMT-B training at Johnson County Hospital, Johnsonville, WA.

Certifications

AHA CPR for Healthcare Providers
ACLS Instructor
PHTLS Instructor
Washington State Paramedic, certificate # 294421
Nationally Registered Paramedic
Washington State EMS Primary Instructor
Firefighter I and Firefighter II

Figure 21-2
Curriculum Vita Format

Curriculum Vita
David Long
68 Cardinal Drive
Champaign, IL 50000
(988) 555-4111
Delong@sgnet.com

Personal Data

Born June 15, 1970, in Monroe, MI
United States citizen

Education

MSEd., Adult Education, Illinois Central University, 2002

BFA, Architecture, Idaho College of Fine Arts, 1993

AAS, Emergency Medical Services, Greater Monroe Community
College, 1990

EMS Primary Instructor, Urbana (IL) Community College, 2000

EMT-B, Millersville Fire Department, Millersville, MI, 1988

Employment

EMS Educator, Urbana (IL) Community College, 2000–present

Paramedic, Monroe (MI) Hospital Ambulance Service, 1990–1991

Paramedic, Part-time, Boise (ID) Ambulance Company, 1991–1993

Design technician, Brothers' Building Design and Construction,
Champaign, IL, 1993–2000

Volunteer Work

EMT-B, Rural Rescue, Nortonville, IL, 1988–1990

Paramedic, Rural Rescue, Nortonville, IL, 1990–1991

Paramedic, Clarkston (ID) Rescue Squad, 1991–1993

Paramedic, Urbana (IL) Rescue, 1993–present

Publication

Long, D. 1999. Keeping ahead of the game: Treating the pediatric
trauma patient. *Atlantic EMS Quarterly* 4(3): 17–24.

Long, D., and L. J. Murford. 2000. Writing ambulance specifications.
Western EMS Monthly 10(2): 34–38.

Research

Allison, B. S., J. T. Worth, and D. Long. 2003. A social interactionist
view of paramedic decision making in resuscitation dilemmas.
Research in EMS 3(7): 143–54.

Association of State EMS Training Coordinators, the National Association of EMS Physicians, NAEMSE, and others either have job postings or have links to job postings.

Answering an Ad

If you are interested in interviewing for a position, send a letter of inquiry to the designated person along with your résumé or CV. Describe in your letter where you saw the ad and why you are interested. Don't repeat what is covered in your CV or résumé, but reference your qualifications in the attached document in a statement such as, "As you will note in my résumé, my educational preparation and work experience make me a good fit with the requirements listed for this job." Don't forget to ask for an interview, state how you can be contacted (even if it is on your CV or résumé), and state that you are looking forward to discussing the opportunity with the addressee. Use a formal business letter format and quality stationery for your letter and envelope. Using a tasteful, light color for your stationery makes your letter and résumé or CV stand out among others.

Interviewing

A job interview is not only your chance to demonstrate how you can be a valuable asset to and meet the needs of the organization, but it is also your opportunity to preview the organization and see if it is a place you want to work. Although the interviewer is ethically obligated to give you a **realistic job preview,** this is not always the case. Be prepared to seek other sources of information about the organization. In addition to the tips here, you can find comprehensive interview-preparation resources on the monster.com Web site.

- Prepare for the interview. Research the organization, evaluate your strengths, and anticipate questions that may be asked and how you will answer them.
- As difficult as it is, relax (as much as possible).
- Avoid stereotyped phrases, and explain things in your own words.
- Anticipate open-ended questions such as, Tell me about yourself, and Tell me about a time when you had to _____.
- Be prepared to talk.
- Arrive several minutes prior to the scheduled time of the interview.
- Men and women should both dress in business attire (suits).
- Turn off your cell phone or pager, or better yet, leave it in your car.
- Bring a copy of your résumé or CV, even if you've already submitted one.
- Make notes about the questions you have and strengths you want to emphasize (and bring them with you).
- Observe the culture of the organization. Are people friendly, relaxed and outgoing, or reserved? How do people dress and interact with each other? What do people's offices say about them? What are the classrooms and labs like?
- Ask how your prospective immediate supervisor prefers to interact with employees. How much latitude will you have in decision making?
- If all the answers you get are "right" but your gut feeling tells you something's not right with the situation, trust your gut instinct.
- After the interview, follow up with a thank-you note or letter.

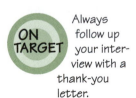

ON TARGET Always follow up your interview with a thank-you letter.

The Job Offer

Assuming the interview (and perhaps a second interview) went well and you're offered the job, should you take it? Consider the positives and negatives of taking the job. Is the work what you want to do? Is there potential for career growth? Do you think you can work for or with the people you met at your interview? Is the salary offered commensurate with your qualifications and experience as well as the work you'll be doing? Are the benefits satisfactory? If you'll be relocating for the job, are relocation expenses reimbursed? And finally, consider that there is wide variability in the cost of living across the country. What might be an adequate salary in the Midwest may leave you unable to meet your financial obligations on the East Coast. There are a variety of salary and relocation calculators on the Internet. They are useful as a guideline but are not 100% accurate, so give yourself a little breathing room.

PEARLS *Don't consider just the job. Consider the employer and the community you'll be in if you take the job.*

Research and Writing for Publication

Participating as an investigator in research projects and writing for publication are two activities that can contribute greatly to your professional appeal. Although most research takes place in universities or larger institutions, writing for publication does not depend upon where you work. If you seek to publish in a newsletter or trade magazine, read several volumes to get a feel for the type of writing published. These publications list guidelines for authors to assist you in the preparation of your article. If you are not proficient in writing for publication, writing workshops are offered at many conferences and faculty development workshops. Once you have honed your presentation skills, you may also want to consider developing a presentation and submitting it for consideration for a professional conference.

Summary

Although it may not seem like it the first few times you stand before a class, teaching is a worthwhile and satisfying activity. In order to be your best and, therefore, increase the satisfaction you derive from teaching, you must engage in a process of lifelong learning, continually striving to enrich the educational experience you provide for your students. Professional development can take place through, but is not limited to, conferences; reading newsletters, trade magazines, and journals; participating in professional organizations; collaborating with peers; and pursuing additional formal education. Beyond this, you can direct your own education through assessing your interests and needs for improvement and seeking out relevant information and activities.

REVIEW QUESTIONS

1. Briefly differentiate between a résumé and curriculum vita.

2. What are some considerations to keep in mind when preparing for or during an interview?

3. Discuss ways of engaging in professional development.

4. Describe the benefits of membership in professional organizations.

References

Chapter 1

Darkenwald, G. G., and S. B. Merriam. 1982. *Adult education: Foundations of practice.* New York: HarperCollins.

National Academy of Sciences National Research Council. 1966. *Accidental death and disability: The neglected disease of modern society.*

NHTSA (National Highway Traffic Safety Administration). 1996. *EMS agenda for the future.*

———. 2000. *EMS education agenda for the future: A systems approach.* Retrieved July 17, 2003, from http://www.nhtsa.dot.gov/people/injury/ems?EdAgenda/final/agenda6-00.htm.

———. 2002. *2002 national guidelines for EMS educators.* Retrieved January 2, 2004, from http://www.nhtsa.dot.gov/people/injury/ems/Instructor/instructor_ems/2002_national_guidelines.htm..

Chapter 2

Argyris, C. 1982. *Reasoning, learning, and action.* San Francisco: Jossey-Bass.

Dewey, J. 1938. *Experience and education.* New York: MacMillan.

Merriam, S. B., and R. S. Caffarella. 1999. *Learning in adulthood: A comprehensive guide,* 2d ed. San Francisco: Jossey-Bass.

NHTSA (National Highway Traffic Safety Administration). 1998. *National standard paramedic curriculum.*

Tisdell, E. J., and E. W. Taylor. 2000. Adult education philosophy informs practice. *Adult Learning* 11(2): 6–10.

Chapter 3

Guthrie, V. L. 1996. The relationship of levels of intellectual development and levels of tolerance for diversity among college students. Unpublished doctoral dissertation, Bowling Green State University, OH.

Kohlberg, L. 1969. Stage and sequence: The cognitive developmental approach to socialization. In *The handbook of socialization theory and research*, ed. D. Goslin. Chicago: Rand McNally.

NHTSA (National Highway Traffic Safety Administration). 1998. Paramedic functional job description. *National Standard Paramedic Curriculum*.

Rest, J. 1984. The major components of morality. In *Morality, moral behavior, and moral development*, ed. W. Kurtines and J. Gewirtz. New York: Wiley.

Chapter 4

Lindstrom, A. and K. Losavio. 2004. JEMS 2004 platinum resource guide. *Journal of Emergency Medical Services* 29: 1.

NHTSA (National Highway Traffic Safety Administration). 1996. *EMS agenda for the future.*

———. 1998. *National standard paramedic curriculum.*

Chapter 5

NHTSA (National Highway Traffic Safety Administration). 2002. *2002 national guidelines for ems educators.* Retrieved January 2, 2004, from http://www.nhtsa.dot.gov/people/injury/ems/Instructor/instructor_ems/2002_national_guidelines.htm.

Chapter 6

Baron, R. A., and J. Greenberg. 2000. *Behavior in organizations*, 7th ed. Upper Saddle River, NJ: Prentice Hall.

Carney, P. 2000. Adult learning styles: implications for practice teaching in social work. *Social Work Education* 19(6): 609–26.

Gardner, H. 1983. *Frames of mind: The theory of multiple intelligences.* New York: Basic Books.

Jones, C., C. Reichard, and K. Mokhtari. 2003. Are students' learning styles discipline specific? *Community College Journal of Research and Practice* 27: 363–75.

Knowles, M. S. (1980). *The modern practice of adult education: From pedagogy to andragogy.* New York: Cambridge Book Co.

Lawrence, G. 1993. *People types and tiger stripes*. Gainesville, FL: The Center for Application of Psychological Types, Inc.

Levinson, D. J., and J. D. Levinson. (1996). *The seasons of a woman's life*. New York: Ballantine.

Merriam, S. B., and R. S. Caffarella. 2000. *Learning in adulthood*, 2d ed. San Francisco: Jossey-Bass.

Severiens, S., G. T. Dam, and E. Nijenhuis. 1998. Ways of knowing and patterns of reasoning: Women and men in adult secondary education. *Gender and Education*, 10(3): 327–42.

Chapter 7

Baddeley, A. 1992. Working memory. *Science* 255: 556–59.

Blanchard, P. N., and J. W. Thacker. 1999. *Effective training: Systems, strategies and practices*. Upper Saddle River, NJ: Prentice Hall.

Bloom, Benjamin S., et al. 1956. *Taxonomy of educational objectives, book I: Cognitive domain*. New York: Longman.

Dewey, J. 1938. *Experience and education*. Kappa Delta Pi Fraternity.

Diamond, M.C. 2002. *Response of the brain to enrichment*. Retrieved 06/08/2003 from http://www.newhorizons.org/neuro/diamond_brain_response.htm.

Houle, C. 1980. *Continuing learning in the professions*. San Francisco: Jossey-Bass.

Howard Hughes Medical Institute. 2002. *A new window to view how experiences rewire the brain*. Retrieved 05/22/2003 from http://www.newhorizons.org/neuro/hhmi.htm.

Jarvis, P. 1995. *Adult and continuing education: Theory and practice*, 2d ed. London: Routledge.

Kivinen, O., and P. Ristela. 2002. Even higher learning takes place by doing: From postmodern critique to pragmatic action. *Studies in Higher Education* 27(4): 419–30.

Sewell, A. 2002. Constructivism and student misconceptions: Why every teacher needs to know about them. *Australian Science Teachers Journal* 48(4): 24–28.

Smith, M. 2001. David A. Kolb on experiential learning. *The encyclopedia of informal education*. Retrieved 06/06/2003 from http://www.infed.org/biblio/b-explrn.htm.

Sweller, J., J. J. G. van Merrienboer, and F. G. W. C. Pass. 1998. Cognitive architecture and instructional design. *Educational Psychology Review* 10(3): 251–96.

Chapter 8

Caffarella, R. S. 1994. *Planning programs for adult learners: A practical guide for educators, trainers and staff developers.* San Francisco: Jossey-Bass.

Dewey, J. 1938. *Experience and education.* New York: MacMillan.

Donaldson, L., and E. E. Scannell. 1986. *Human resources development: The new trainer's guide,* 2d ed. Reading, MA: Addison-Wesley.

Gable, K. E. 1980. An interpretation of Tyler's model of curriculum development. Unpublished.

Mager, R. F., and P. Pipe. 1997. *Analyzing performance problems, or you really oughta wanna: How to figure out why people aren't doing what they should be, and what to do about it,* 3d ed. Atlanta: The Center for Effective Performance, Inc.

NHTSA. 1998. *National standard paramedic curriculum.*

NREMT. 2005. Retrieved March 30 2005, from www.NREMT.org/about/about_exams.asp

Prideaux, D. 2003. ABC of learning and teaching in medicine: Curriculum design. *British Medical Journal* (326): 268–370.

Seibert, M. L. 1979. Establishing criteria for competency-based education. *American Journal of Medical Technology,* 45(5): 368–71.

Tyler, R. W. 1949. *Basic principles of curriculum and instruction.* Chicago: The University of Chicago Press.

Chapter 9

Donaldson, L., and E. E. Scannell. 1986. *Human resources development: The new trainer's guide,* 2d ed. Reading, MA: Addison-Wesley Publishers.

Harvey, R. J. 1991. Job analysis. In *Handbook of industrial and organizational psychology,* 2d ed., ed. M. Dunnette and L Hought. Palo Alto, CA: Consulting Psychologists Press.

Militello, L. G., and R. J. B. Hutton. 1998. Applied cognitive task analysis (ACTA): A practitioner's toolkit for understanding cognitive task demands. *Ergonomics* 41(11): 1618–1641.

NHTSA (National Highway Traffic Safety Administration). 1998. *National standard paramedic curriculum.*

Raymond, M. R. 2001. Job analysis and the specification of content for licensure and certification examinations. *Applied Measurement in Education* 14(4): 369–415.

Chapter 12

Caffarella, R.S. 1994. *Planning programs for adult learners: A practical guide for educators, trainers and staff developers.* San Francisco: Jossey-Bass.

Donaldson, L., and E. E. Scannell. 1986. *Human resource development: The new trainer's guide,* 2d ed. Reading, MA: Addison-Wesley Publishers.

Koon, J., and H. G. Murray. 1995. Using multiple outcomes to validate student ratings of overall teacher effectiveness. *The Journal of Higher Education* 66(1): 61–72.

Chapter 13

Gronlund, N. E. 1993. *How to make achievement tests and assessments,* 5th ed. Boston: Allyn and Bacon.

Chapter 14

Alexander, M., D. Limmer, and K. Monosky. 2002. The horns and halo effect: Examining preceptor bias in preceptor evaluation of student performance. Abstract. *Prehospital Emergency Care* 6(2, October).

Baron, R. A., and J. Greenberg. 2000. *Behavior in organizations,* 7th ed. Upper Saddle River, NJ: Prentice Hall.

Gronlund, N. E. 1993. *How to make achievement tests and assessments,* 5th ed. Boston: Allyn and Bacon.

Chapter 18

Archer, J., and J. J. Schevak. 1998. Enhancing students' motivation to learn: Achievement goals in university classrooms. *Educational Psychology* 18(2): 205–23.

Chory-Assad, R. M. 2002. Classroom justice: Perceptions of fairness as a predictor of student motivation, learning, and aggression. *Communication Quarterly* 50(1): 58–77.

Donaldson, L., and E. E. Scannell. 1986. *Human resource development: The new trainer's guide,* 2d ed. Reading, MA: Addison-Wesley.

Greenberg, J., and R. A. Baron. 2000. *Behavior in organizations,* 7th ed. Upper Saddle River, NJ: Prentice Hall.

Mager, R. F., and P. Pipe. 1997. *Analyzing performance problems,* 3d ed. Atlanta, GA: The Center for Effective Performance.

Maslow, A. H. 1943. A theory of human motivation. *Psychological Review* 50: 370–96.

McClincy, W. D. 1995. *Instructional methods in emergency services.* Upper Saddle River, NJ: Brady Prentice Hall.

McKeachie, W. J. 1994. *Teaching tips: Strategies, research and theory for college and university teachers,* 9th ed. Lexington, MA: D. C. Heath.

Parvensky, C. A. 1995. *Teaching EMS: An educator's guide to improved EMS instruction.* St. Louis: Mosby.

Chapter 19

Dave, R. 1967. *Psychomotor domain.* Berlin: International Conference of Educational Testing.

George, J. H., and F. X. Doto. 2001. A simple five-step method for teaching clinical skills. *Family Medicine* 33(8): 577–78.

Harrelson, G. L., and D. Leaver-Dunn. 2002. Using the experiential learning cycle in clinical instruction. *Athletic Therapy Today* 7(5): 23–27.

McClincy, W. D. 1995. *Instructional methods in emergency services.* Upper Saddle River, NJ: Prentice Hall.

Moore, M. L., and J. F. Perry. 1976. *Clinical education in physical therapy: Present status/future needs. Final Report of the Project on Clinical Education in Physical Therapy.* New York: American Physical Therapy Association.

Polanyi, M. 1966. *The tacit dimension.* Garden City, NY: Doubleday.

Romiszowski, A. 2004. *Instruction in the psychomotor domain.* Retreived May 12, 2004 from http://www.personal.psu.edu/users/j/u/jux100/PS-%20main%20page.htm.

Schön, D. A. 1987. *Educating the reflective practitioner.* San Francisco: Jossey-Bass.

Seibert, M. L. 1979. Establishing criteria for competency-based education. *American Journal of Medical Technology* 45(5): 368–71.

Simpson, E. 1972. *The classification of educational objectives in the psychomotor domain: The psychomotor domain,* vol. 3. Washington, DC: Gryphon House.

Chapter 20

CoAEMSP (Committee on Accreditation of Education Programs for the Emergency Medical Services Professions). 1999. *Standards and guidelines.* Retrieved June 14, 2004, from http://www.coaemsp.org/standardspolicies.htm.

Further Reading

Chapter 2

Elias, J. L., and S. B. Merriam. 1980. *Philosophical foundations of adult education*. Malabar, FL: Krieger Publishing Co.

Merriam, S. B., and R. G. Brockett. 1997. *The profession and practice of adult education: an introduction*. San Francisco: Jossey-Bass.

Price, D. W. 2000. Philosophy and the adult educator. *Adult Learning* 11(2): 3–5.

Chapter 3

Branch, W. T. 2001. Supporting the moral development of medical students. *Journal of General Internal Medicine* 15: 503–8.

Mathiasen, R. E. 1998. Moral education of college students: Faculty and staff perspectives. *College Student Journal* 32(3): 374–77.

McKeachie, W. J. 1994. *Teaching values: Should we? Can we?*, 9th ed. Lexington, MA: DC Heath & Co., 373–84.

Morgan, B., F. Morgan, V. Foster, and J. Kolbert. 2000. Promoting the moral and conceptual development of law enforcement trainees: A deliberate psychological educational approach. *Journal of Moral Education* 29(2): 203–18.

Chapter 4

Caffarella, R. S. 1994. *Planning programs for adult learners: A practical guide for educators, trainers, and staff developers*. San Francisco: Jossey-Bass.

Chapter 5

Apps, J. W. 1994. *Leadership for the emerging age: Transforming practice in adult and continuing education*. San Francisco: Jossey-Bass.

McKeachie, W. J. 1994. *Teaching tips: strategies, research, and theory for college and university teachers*, 9th ed. Lexington, MA: DC Heath and Co.

Chapter 6

Datan, N., D. Rodeheaver, and F. Hughes. 1987. Adult development and aging. *Annual Review of Psychology* 38: 153–80.

Moran, J. J. 1990. Promoting cognitive development through adult education. *Education* 112(2): 186–94.

Chapter 7

Howard Hughes Medical Institute. 2002. *A new window to view how experiences rewire the brain.* Retrieved 05/22/2003 from http://www.newhorizons.org/neuro/hhmi.htm.

Chapter 8

Caffarella, R. S. 1994. *Planning programs for adult learners: A practical guide for educators, trainers and staff developers.* San Francisco: Jossey-Bass.

Donaldson, L., and E. E. Scannell. 1986. *Human resources development: The new trainer's guide,* 2d ed. Reading, MA: Addison-Wesley Publishers.

Mager, R. F., and P. Pipe. 1997. *Analyzing performance problems, or you really oughta wanna: How to figure out why people aren't doing what they should be, and what to do about it,* 3d ed. Atlanta: The Center for Effective Performance, Inc.

Chapter 9

Denis, J., and B. Austin. 1992. A BASE(ic) course on job analysis. *Training and Development* (July): 67–70.

Donaldson, L., and Scannell, E. E. 1986. *Human resources development: The new trainer's guide,* 2nd ed. Reading, MA: Addison-Wesley.

Chapter 10

Bloom, B. S. 1956. *Taxonomy of educational objectives, book I: Cognitive domain.* New York: Longman.

Chapter 12

Caffarella, R. S. 1994. *Planning programs for adult learners: A practical guide for educators, trainers and staff developers.* San Francisco: Jossey-Bass.

Donaldson, L., and E. E. Scannell. (1986). *Human resource development: The new trainer's guide,* 2d ed. Reading, MA: Addison-Wesley Publishers.

McKeachie, W. J. 1994. *Teaching tips: Strategies, research and theory for college and university teachers,* 9th ed. Lexington, MA: D.C. Heath and Co.

Murray, H. G. (1983). Low interference classroom teaching behaviors and student ratings of college teaching effectiveness. *Journal of Educational Psychology* 75: 138–49.

Sources of Sample Teaching-Effectiveness Questions

http://www.wmich.edu/teachlearn/new/self_eval_tch.htm

http://www/education.mcgill.ca/cutl/tendimen.html

Chapter 13

Colorado State University Writing Guide:
http://writing.colostate.edu/references/research/relval/com2a5.cfm.

Gronlund, N. E. 1993. *How to make achievement tests and assessments,* 5th ed. Boston: Allyn and Bacon.

McKeachie, W. J. 1994. *Teaching tips: strategies, research, and theory for college and university teachers,* 9th ed. Lexington, MA: D.C. Heath.

Popham, W. J. 1995. *Classroom assessment: What teachers need to know.* Boston: Allyn and Bacon.

Chapter 16

Blanchard, P. N., and J. W. Thacker. 1999. *Effective training: Systems, strategies and practices.* Upper Saddle River, NJ: Prentice Hall.

Donaldson, L., and E. E. Scannell. 1986. *Human resource development: The new trainer's guide,* 2d ed. Reading, MA: Addison-Wesley.

Chapter 17

Blanchard, P. N., and J. W. Thacker. 1999. *Effective training: Systems, strategies, and practices.* Upper Saddle River, NJ: Prentice Hall.

Bligh, D. A. 2000. *What's the use of lectures.* San Francisco: Jossey-Bass.

McKeachie, W. J. 1994. *Teaching tips: Strategies, research and theory for college and university teachers,* 9th ed. Lexington, MA: D. C. Heath.

Chapter 18

Archer, J., and J. J. Schevak. 1998. Enhancing students' motivation to learn: Achievement goals in university classrooms. *Educational Psychology* 18(2): 205–23.

Chory-Assad, R. M. 2002. Classroom justice: perceptions of fairness as a predictor of student motivation, learning, and aggression. *Communication Quarterly* 50(1): 58–77.

Maslow, A. H. 1943. A theory of human motivation. *Psychological Review* 50: 370–96.

Answers to
Case Study Questions

Chapter 1

1. Ben and Trey have more options available to them for paramedic education than ever before. Because Ben will need at least a bachelor's degree to meet his career goals, he may want to attend a certificate or associate's degree paramedic program in a community college and then transfer to a university to finish his bachelor's degree, or he may elect to attend a university program from the start. Although Trey certainly has these options as well, he could also elect to attend a hospital-based program if he does not wish to obtain academic credit for his program.

2. Things have changed tremendously in EMS education in the past 25 years. In addition to the increased number of choices for EMS education, curriculum-development processes have continuously improved and EMS students can now receive academic credit for their studies. It is now much more likely that a student has an accredited program in his or her area to help ensure program adherence to educational standards.

3. Ben and Trey should expect that their instructors are competent in instruction. In addition to asking about the academic credentials of their potential instructors, they will also want to know whether their instructors have accomplished the competencies expected of EMS educators, as listed by NAEMSE.

Chapter 2

1. The students do not seem familiar with taking an active role in their learning but instead seem to think that having the written notes and slides will be an effective way for them to learn. This expectation for passive reception of information is most consistent with liberal education.

2. Rita is trying to get the students to ask questions and actively participate in discussions based on case studies. She knows that passively receiving the information is not an effective way to learn. This is most consistent with progressive information.

3. Anne might point out that it is not uncommon for students to come into the classroom with different expectations for the teaching-learning transaction than those of the instructor. She could advise Anne that it might be helpful to share

her perspectives on learning with her next class from the very beginning, explaining to them how actively using the information in class is much more effective than just reading someone's notes on it.

Chapter 3

Such situations are always stressful for instructors. Clear and inclusive course policies and impartiality in dealing with students is essential to minimizing such complaints, but even in the best of circumstances, disappointed students may have a very different perspective on what is right and wrong. Giving and documenting student feedback and counseling sessions, as well as getting students' written acknowledgment of receipt of policies and procedures, are important ways of minimizing liability.

1. It appears that there were program policies in place to guide Neil's decisions and that Neil followed the policies. Jim's shortcomings in dynamic cardiology were noted by the initial skills' evaluator and the medical director, as well as by Neil. As long as the policies have been applied fairly and consistently by the program, Jim's request does not appear appropriate.

2. Jim's overall academic performance establishes a pattern of marginal achievement. His failure of the practical exam station does not represent a significant departure from his usual performance. Course policies were in place and were followed, and Jim's performance was witnessed by multiple observers.

3. Although we cannot be sure of the manner in which it was delivered, a statement of the actual outcome of a proposed treatment, in this case the patient's death, is not intimidation. Neil has an obligation to correct errors in the laboratory.

4. The program has an ethical obligation to treat students fairly. The program also has an ethical obligation to the public and to other health-care providers to uphold standards of performance. Michelle has an ethical obligation to support Neil's decision, if the facts show that Neil was fair and followed program policies. Jim, although he apparently doesn't recognize it, has an ethical (and moral) obligation to "do no harm" to his potential patients. By insisting that he retest without proper remediation, he could conceivably have a "good day" and marginally pass the test, although he is not likely to perform competently in the field under those circumstances.

Chapter 4

1. In addition to her instructor certificate, Maria might be expected to hold instructor cards in a variety of specialty courses, such as CPR, ACLS, PHTLS, and PALS.

2. To work in a community college program, Maria is likely to need a minimum of an associate's degree, and possibly a bachelor's degree. She also may need to be licensed as a community college instructor in her state.

3. In some states, vocational educators must hold the same secondary teaching license as other faculty, but in others there is a different process for vocational teacher licensing. Maria may need to complete additional course work and/or take a licensure examination.

Chapter 5

1. As a primary instructor, Todd will have increased responsibilities for course planning, coordination, and evaluation. The exact roles and responsibilities will vary from institution to institution, but Todd is likely to be responsible for filling out administrative paperwork, seeking involvement from the course medical director, managing the course schedule, student assignments and testing, and arranging for guest instructors.
2. Todd will be expected to have more responsibility and should make sure that his compensation reflects this. He will want to determine if the expectations for responsibility are reasonable. Among the several things that Todd will want to ask Pam about include the exact roles and responsibilities of the position, the number of hours in the classroom, how much time he will have for administrative and coordination functions, and whether he will be responsible for coordinating and supervising other instructional staff.
3. All instructors should strive to demonstrate integrity and honesty, be empathetic and compassionate, self-motivated, professional in appearance, self-confident, and able to communicate clearly, make effective use of time, be an advocate of teamwork, be diplomatic and respectful in interactions with others, value lifelong learning, be knowledgeable about the subject matter being taught, and be an advocate for the student.

Chapter 6

There are a number of motivational, situational, developmental, and personality factors behind people's behavior. We can consider personality traits such as extraversion and intraversion, the assumptions of androgogy concerning the needs of adult learners, learning styles, and theories of motivation, as well as cultural differences. Understanding these factors is helpful both in determining possible reasons for behavior and in finding solutions to the resulting situations.

1. Tom may have learned much of the course material through experience. Calling on Tom's experience during class and lab will provide a learning opportunity for the other students and will keep Tom more engaged in the class.
2. Although Andy and J. T. do not seem to have a primary interest in EMS, they are apparently motivated by promotional opportunities. By relating success in the course to increased potential for promotion, these students are more likely to increase their effort in the course. Most adults also have a deep need to feel competent in their work. This is another way of appealing to Andy and J. T.

3. Although there could be a number of things behind Betsey's behavior, one thing to consider is that she may not otherwise have much of an opportunity to socialize and that talking in class helps her meet the need to socialize. Betsey is also probably very extraverted and doesn't realize she is monopolizing class time. One way of handling this is to call on her less often in class. Specific ways of handling talkative students are discussed in Chapter 18. If she continues, it may ultimately be necessary to speak with her outside of class.

4. Robert may be introverted and easily annoyed by unnecessary talkativeness. He seems to have a straightforward problem-centered reason for being in the class. He is in the class to learn more skills for his job and may not see the relevance of Betsey's personal stories.

Chapter 7

1. Danielle should consider arranging the material to begin with what is already in the students' experience. For example, if her class has already discussed anatomy and physiology, she can begin from that point. She will want to sequence from simple to more complex, as well.

2. Danielle will want to keep in mind the limitations of working memory so that students are not receiving information so quickly that they cannot process it. She should also consider the clarity of her message so she does not add extrinsic cognitive load to the inherent difficulty of the material. Because experience can often provide a platform for further learning, Danielle may want to present essential material, have the students learn the skills, and then have a more in-depth discussion with students, allowing them to draw from their lab experiences.

3. Based on what Danielle has expressed as her goals for her students, she will want to write objectives in all three domains of learning: affective, cognitive, and psychomotor.

Chapter 8

Education and training are often thought to be remedies for problems that are not caused by a lack of knowledge or skill. Before developing an educational program, the first step is to determine if the problem is one of knowledge or skill deficit.

1. It is unclear from the information given whether the failure to successfully intubate the trauma patient resulted from inadequate knowledge or skill. More information is needed.

2. One way to determine if education is required is to use the Mager analysis. This is a systematic way of determining what factors lead to the problem. For example, the patient was successfully intubated after receiving RSI. Did paramedic Davies have this option available to him? Perhaps he did not have the resources needed to care for that patient. Has paramedic Davies failed to intubate other patients? Under what conditions?

3. This situation might require a change in protocol or perhaps a change in expectations if the protocol is not revised. There may be a number of ways of providing paramedics in this agency with an increased number of options for dealing with difficult airway situations.

Chapter 9

1. Jillian's first step is to conduct a systematic needs analysis to determine where training should be targeted.
2. Jillian will need to find out what the critical tasks and knowledge are for the employees. Critical-care transport requires skills and knowledge not commonly used by many EMTs and paramedics. She will need to determine what kinds of patients are transported by the service, how long their transport times are, what kinds of issues arise for the employees, and any known concerns of employees and management.
3. Jillian can conduct surveys and interviews of employees and management, or she can ride along with the service for a few shifts, conduct performance testing, and ask for CQI findings.
4. Jillian should prepare a formal training proposal stating her findings and recommendations, the probable outcomes with and without training, and the time and costs involved.

Chapter 10

1. The general competencies related to recognizing and managing poisoning patients have been established in the NSC. Danny can use these as a starting place. The needs analysis revealed a specific local need for information and Danny must integrate this information into his objectives. Danny will use the competencies as terminal performance objectives and will use information from the needs assessment to build enabling objectives to meet the needs of his audience.
2. Danny will need to consider that he will be building his lesson plan and evaluation tools from these objectives.
3. By asking himself, What is it I really want the attendees to be able to do? Danny will be able to select appropriate verbs to describe the behavior.

Chapter 11

This is an exciting opportunity for Barbara, but being a new primary instructor, she could use some guidance.

1. Barbara should find out what the concerns are about the current format and any limitations or assumptions that Janie has about the program format.
2. Barbara could either make changes but keep a one-semester program, or she might consider a two-semester program or a summer-session course.

3. Most states and/or institutions have formulas for assigning credit hours, so Barbara must find out what the ratio of clock hours to credit hours is at this institution.

4. Barbara needs to consider how the program is impacted by state regulatory guidelines and institutional guidelines.

Chapter 12

1. Because there appear to be no written or electronic records of program performance, Ty will need to collect some data of his own. He might be able to access program-testing statistics from the state regulatory agency or the National Registry of EMTs. He could interview or survey current and former students, field training officers, and supervisors. He could also follow up with any paramedic programs that may have admitted EMTs who completed the program.

2. Ty could ask for reports on exam statistics, create online or paper questionnaires, or design an interview protocol to collect the information in a uniform manner.

3. The first step in getting back on track is to diagnose the problem. Once the problem has been diagnosed, the root causes of the problems should be sought, goals established, and an action plan devised.

4. Ty must build benchmarks and criteria into an evaluation plan based on the action-plan goals. He will need to establish methods and a schedule for assessment and revise the action plan accordingly.

5. Ongoing program evaluation and revision is the key to detecting and correcting problems in a timely manner.

Chapter 13

1. The best way to ensure that an exam accurately represents course material is to create a table of exam specifications.

2. It's premature to say whether Shelly should adjust the scoring in any way. Even if some things were not represented on the exam, if the items on the exam were "fair game" from the objectives, then students should be expected to know the information. If there are, indeed, a couple of bad test items, Shelly can address those items by either dropping them from the exam or accepting more than one correct answer for those items.

3. When Shelly reviews the items in retrospect, it may become clear to her what the students are complaining about. Often, a question we think is written clearly doesn't seem to be later on when we come back to it in a different frame of mind. This can often be prevented by having another instructor read the exam items before making a final version of the exam. If the question is not obviously flawed, Shelly should ask the complaining students to put their concerns in writing with a reference to information that supports their case.

Chapter 14

1. Multiple-choice items, like all selection items, are best suited for evaluating lower-level learning outcomes. Although higher-level learning outcomes can be evaluated with multiple-choice items, the construction of this type of item is time consuming and difficult.

2. Multiple-choice items are objective and easy to grade but somewhat difficult to write in a manner that ensures measurement of the true competencies of interest. It is possible for students to guess the correct answer, but this tendency is decreased by using attractive and plausible distracters.

3. Depending upon the objectives John wants to measure, he could use matching, true/false, short-answer, and restricted-response essay items on his test. Short-answer and fill-in-the-blank-type items are generally easier to write than multiple-choice items. The probability of students guessing correctly is high for true/false items, but students can bluff on supply-type items. These types of items can all be acceptable if guidelines for constructing them are followed.

Chapter 15

1. There are a number of considerations in determining which equipment should be purchased. Even in the ideal circumstance, in which money is no object and all requests could financially be accommodated, purchases must still be made wisely. Micki will need to know at least the following:

   a. Is this equipment to meet a new perceived need, or is it to replace existing equipment?

   b. If it is a new perceived need, how has this need been determined? Can it be justified? What would be the result of not purchasing the item?

   c. If this is to replace existing equipment, is this a regularly scheduled replacement, or is the item being replaced sooner than expected? If the item is being replaced sooner than expected, why? Was it not as durable as it was expected to be? Is it under warranty? Can it be repaired? What is the cost of repair compared to the cost of replacement? If it is a regularly scheduled replacement, is the item being replaced while it is still useful? If so, can the item be traded in or donated, or should it be kept and replacement deferred?

2. Once Micki has decided which items should be purchased, she needs to see how the requests fit into the equipment budget. She needs to price the items and, potentially, prioritize them. Sources of information include information obtained from trade shows and professional journals, equipment vendor catalogs, and sales representatives. Micki should look at alternative models for each item and their advantages and limitations against their initial cost and potential costs of maintenance. She needs to consider warranties and maintenance contracts as well as in-house resources for maintenance and repair.

Chapter 16

1. This presents a dilemma for Manny. If his colleague is accustomed to teaching trauma topics and is well versed in the material, the colleague's lesson plans may not include sufficient detail for Manny to feel comfortable teaching from them. If he chooses to use his colleague's materials, he will still need to research the topics and create his own notes. A commercially prepared lesson plan would be convenient, as well, but would also require Manny to research the topics and adapt the lesson plan to suit his needs. Creating his own lesson plan is an option, too. Manny will need to consider how closely each option meets his needs and time lines.

2. Manny will need to begin by obtaining the objectives and reading the student text. He will then need to do additional research to ensure that he is familiar with the content beyond the level expected of the students. If possible, he will want to talk with his colleague to see what information and activities the colleague typically uses that might not appear in the lesson plan.

Chapter 17

1. Latrice might consider starting with a case study to attract students' attention, or she might use a simulation or demonstration involving age-related changes in the senses. Although demonstration and simulation are often thought of as laboratory activities, they would be quite appropriate in this situation. Nearly everyone has some experience with the elderly. This fact provides Latrice with the opportunity to facilitate a discussion that incorporates students' experiences.

2. Some possible questions include, What are some significant ways in which the elderly are different than younger adults? Why do you think it's important for us to discuss the elderly as a group with specific considerations and needs? What are some of the stereotypes that people hold about the elderly? What is the impact of people holding these stereotypes about the elderly?

3. Games and CBI are probably not ideally suited for this particular group and purpose, although CBI might be used as a supplemental activity.

4. The most important way for Latrice to help reduce her anxiety is for her to be well prepared in order to increase her confidence. This includes knowing her audience and her topic. Providing activities has the added benefits of taking some of the responsibility for the class off Latrice and placing it on the students and allowing for some physical activity. Her confidence will increase more with experience.

Chapter 18

1. Maslow's hierarchy of needs probably provides the most insight into Bart's behavior. He seems to be driven by social needs and the need for recognition. Regardless of the motivation, the behavior is disruptive and must be addressed.

2. This issue might be particularly difficult to address because Bart cannot see the effect of his behavior on others. It is also difficult to establish the line between appropriate class contribution and overenthusiastic class contribution, so it will be difficult to set criteria for Bart's behavior.

3. In this case, it might be helpful to assist Bart in developing some insight into his behavior. One way is to talk with him and tell him you appreciate the fact that he contributes to class but that he may not be aware that he is preventing others from contributing to class. You might then ask him what he feels the impact is on the class when not everyone is allowed to contribute. You could then explain to Bart that it is your job to ensure that everyone has an opportunity to contribute in class. It might also be helpful to allow students to anonymously evaluate each other's affective behaviors by designing an instrument on which students can rate their classmates' professional characteristics. It is important to emphasize that you are seeking honest feedback, but that the feedback must be professional and designed to help individuals develop professionally.

Chapter 19

1. Most likely, Dave will need to keep records that document student eligibility for clinical participation, such as student certificates, CPR cards, and verification that health status and immunizations are on file, as well as keeping track of student clinical hours, competencies, and preceptor evaluations.

2. Dave will need to review the clinical affiliation agreements with each clinical site. If the specifics of the relationship are not clear, Dave will need to make contact with the site liaison to establish procedures.

3. Dave will need to consider the capacity of the clinical sites, availability of preceptors, and the point at which students are in the curriculum.

4. Dave should expect that preceptors are competent clinicians, are positive role models, are willing to teach and mentor, and have attended a clinical education workshop to develop skills in clinical education and evaluation.

Chapter 20

1. University presidents or chancellors usually report to the university board of directors. Vice presidents and provosts generally report to the president or chancellor, and deans generally report to vice presidents or provosts.

2. In terms of faculty rank, generally the entry level is assistant instructor or professor, followed by associate, full instructor or professor, and professor emeritus. Adjunct or affiliate faculty generally teach a specific course under contract and do not have a regular employment relationship with the university or college. Clinical instructors or professors generally do not teach classes but mentor students or residents in the clinical setting or act as precepts.

3. Support personnel are generally underrecognized and overutilized. They should be treated with respect and with regard for their overall workload, not just the work you would like them to do. Show appreciation for their efforts by remembering administrative assistants' day.

Chapter 21

1. Ed can look for employment opportunities listed in EMS-specific publications—both print and electronic. He should also visit professional association Web sites. If he is not a member of a professional association, he should join at least one now. By doing so, he will add value to his credentials and can participate in listservs that send out information about employment opportunities. Ed can also talk to colleagues about his plan. Word of mouth is a powerful way of putting job seekers and employers together.
2. If Ed is unfamiliar with putting together a résumé or CV, he may want to work with a consultant to help him develop his document. At the very least, he should use a standard format and résumé paper and must carefully proofread his document.
3. The interview is a chance for Ed not only to sell himself to a potential employer, but also to find out if the employer is right for him. He should find out about the stability and direction of the program, plans for the position for which he is interviewing, the organizational structure, and the organizational culture, at a minimum.

Answers to
Review Questions

Chapter 1

1. The 1966 "White Paper," *Accidental Death and Disability: The Neglected Disease of Modern Society*.
2. *The EMS Agenda for the Future* and *The EMS Education Agenda for the Future*.
3. NAEMSE, the National Association of EMS Educators.
4. Adults have more experience, which may either facilitate or act as a barrier to further learning but which must be acknowledged.
5. Refer to the list of competencies on pp. 9–10.

Chapter 2

1. Humanism
2. Constructivist
3. Behaviorism

Chapter 3

1. These can include educational malpractice, student injury, patient injury, harassment, discrimination, and violations of ADA and FERPA, as well as copyright infringement and plagiarism.
2. Educational malpractice occurs when an educator does not follow the standards of educational practice expected of EMS educators, resulting in an adverse outcome.
3. In certain cases, portions of student records can be released with the student's written consent. For example, some students may give permission for an employer to review their grades for the purposes of tuition benefit or reimbursement.
4. A student requesting accommodations under ADA must provide, in advance, documentation of his or her disability.
5. Moral sensitivity refers to an individual's ability to detect moral or ethical elements in a situation.

Chapter 4

1. Law-enforcement academies, fire and rescue academies, secondary schools, government agencies, community colleges, colleges, universities, hospitals, ambulance services.
2. Continuing education content goes beyond the content of preservice education, whereas refresher education reemphasizes the content of preservice education.
3. Community colleges exist to allow widespread and relatively inexpensive access to higher education. They may offer certificates and associate's degrees as well as continuing education. Colleges offer 4-year undergraduate degrees, and universities offer both undergraduate and graduate degrees and emphasize research.
4. There may be state licensing requirements to teach in secondary, vocational, and community college settings, and many employers require instructor certification in specialty courses. It is generally required that the instructor has achieved one educational level higher than that offered by the program in which he or she is teaching.
5. Didactic education generally refers to classroom teaching activities such as lecture, lecture-discussion, and case studies. Laboratory education focuses on learning and practicing skills and integrated scenarios, and clinical education focuses on supervised performance of job tasks in the actual work setting.

Chapter 5

1. The primary distinction between primary and secondary EMS instructors is generally the degree of experience as an instructor. As such, the primary instructor has course administrative roles and responsibilities in addition to teaching-related roles and responsibilities.
2. Integrity, honesty, empathy, compassion, self-motivation, professional appearance, self-confidence, clarity in communications, effective management of time, advocating teamwork, diplomacy, respectfulness, valuing life-long learning, knowledgeable of the subject matter being taught, and an advocate for the student.
3. Who the audience is, what the relationship is with the audience, employer practices and policies, and whether the class involves lecture or skills.
4. Preparing lesson plans and tests, conducting lecture and skill sessions.
5. There are many ways in which instructors can act as student advocates. Some examples include facilitating clinical experiences and bringing in potential employers.
6. There are ten competencies of the EMS educator. The EMS educator
   - Understands the concepts and tools of inquiry of the profession.
   - Understands adult learning.
   - Understands learning styles.

- Promotes higher-order thinking and problem solving.
- Understands motivation.
- Uses effective communication.
- Plans and delivers instruction.
- Plans and implements evaluation.
- Engages in reflective practice.
- Cultivates professional relationships.

Chapter 6

1. During middle adulthood, generally age 40 to 65, individuals struggle with stagnation versus generativity.
2. The concrete operational stage is characterized by an either-or orientation and by a lack of tolerance for ambiguity, and there is an inability to consider multiple variables in a situation.
3. The six assumptions of andragogy are
   - Adults need to know why they need to learn something.
   - Adults need to be perceived as self-directing.
   - Adults have an increased quantity and quality of experiences.
   - Adults are ready to learn to cope with immediate life concerns.
   - Adults are problem-centered learners.
   - Adults are intrinsically motivated.
4. The theory of multiple intelligences helps explain why one student learns readily in the classroom but not as readily in lab. It helps to explain why some students are clinically competent but don't have good "people skills," and it helps explain why people are capable of differing degrees of insight about themselves.
5. Expectancy theory.
6. Some suggestions are asking each student to bring in a personal artifact or two and discuss them with the class or asking questions about holidays and cultural differences in showing respect.

Chapter 7

1. The view of constructionism is that we are active builders of our own knowledge. As we take in new information, we compare it to our existing cognitive structures (schemata) and either accept, modify, or reject the information, or modify the existing schema.
2. This is a cognitive objective. In this case, we are not interested in whether the learner hand writes, uses a computer, or dictates the information; we are interested in whether the learner has the knowledge needed to conceptualize the exam.

3. All learning occurs as a result of experience. A world without experiences would be a void with no stimuli to process and so no learning could occur. To have the most impact, experiences are connected in some way to prior experiences, can be linked to future experiences, and lead to reflection and the creation of meaning.
4. The affective domain refers to the moral, ethical, and emotional aspect of learning. The cognitive domain refers to knowledge and thinking processes, and the psychomotor domain refers to kinesthetic skills.
5. Some important ways of stimulating learners to reflect are to ask provocative questions and assign short directed journaling assignments.

Chapter 8

1. Prescriptive curricula are very detailed, containing specific objectives to direct education. Descriptive curricula are more general, providing the context and considerations for education, allowing more latitude on the part of educators.
2. Informal interviews, formal interviews, surveys, performance tests, reports from supervisors, observation of workers, CQI records, formal research, advisory committees.
3. The objectives cannot be developed before determining the nature of the problem but must be determined before deciding on teaching methods, how much time will be involved, evaluation techniques, etc.
4. Program purpose and goals, a philosophy statement, the population to be served, curriculum overview, course titles and descriptions, terminal performance objectives, faculty credentials, required clinical affiliations, advisory committee, accreditation, budget, and references.
5. Curriculum competencies should be derived from job or occupational analyses or practice analyses.

Chapter 9

1. Collecting data to describe verifiable job behaviors performed by workers, including both the tasks performed and the technologies used to accomplish the end results and determining verifiable characteristics of the job context.
2. Task analyses help instructors become aware again of elements of skills that they have been performing unconsciously. By increasing their awareness, instructors are better able to communicate the elements of the task to the learners.
3. The purpose of educational needs analysis is to determine the gap between desired and actual performance in order to target training where it is needed.
4. The objective of the training, what the need for the training is and how this was determined, who the target audience is, the expected outcome with training and without training, how the outcomes will be evaluated, resources needed, timing of the training, benefits of the training, and costs involved.

Chapter 10

1. Goals are broad statements about what the program wants to achieve. Competencies are statements of the primary tasks of a job, and objectives represent the skills and knowledge necessary to attain the competency.
2. Objectives specify not only the content and sequence of the lesson, but also inform the selection of teaching-learning activities.
3. Assessment of learning must be based on what it is the student is expected to do according to the behaviors called for in the objectives.
4. Choosing the precise verb to describe the behavior of interest is important in determining what is to be taught, how it should be taught, and how it should be evaluated. Objectives must describe what we really want the learner to be able to do.
5. A competency states the behavior expected, under what conditions it is to be performed, and the degree or criterion with which it will be measured.

Chapter 11

1. A semester-based format provides a framework for structuring the program but may be a disadvantage when trying to fit a program of predetermined length into a semester. One semester may not be enough time, and two semesters may be too much.
2. A course syllabus should contain the title and number (if in an academic setting) of the course, a course description, goal(s), objectives, and credit hours (if applicable). The syllabus should include the instructor's contact information; address course policies, grading, student obligations, testing, and reading assignments; and include a course schedule.
3. Often, programs are compressed into a shorter schedule for competitive reasons. People often want things as fast as possible, and EMS certifications are no exception. Beyond a certain point, though, the quality of instruction and the ability of the students to learn are compromised by the intensity of the program. Although competition with other programs is a reality in many settings, quality of education must not be sacrificed.

Chapter 12

1. Program prerequisites and entry requirements, recruitment and admissions, marketing, faculty instructional effectiveness, student advising, program goals, curricular sequence and structure, course objectives and content, textbooks and learning resources, classroom and lab facilities, instructional materials, cognitive evaluation procedures, psychomotor evaluation procedures, affective evaluation procedures, clinical education, program-completion rate, certification/national registry exam-pass rates, graduate competence, graduate employment rate.
2. Evaluation must be planned for during the program-planning process.

3. Formative evaluation takes place while the program or course is ongoing; summative evaluation takes place at the end of the program or course.

4. Formal evaluations consist of questionnaires, surveys, interviews, examinations, testing results, etc.; and informal evaluation consists of conversations, looking for puzzled expressions on students' faces, practice quizzes or practical exams, etc.

5. Diagnostic evaluation occurs prior to educational intervention to establish the preexisting level of knowledge and skills so that educational efforts can be appropriately directed.

6. Participant learning, participant reaction, program goals (outcomes).

7. One such example might be failure to pretest. It would not be clear if posttest scores were due to the educational program or if participants already had the knowledge at the beginning of the program.

Chapter 13

1. Norm-referenced evaluation uses the group to which an individual belongs as a point of reference for measurement. It is a measurement relative to the performance of the rest of the group. Criterion-referenced evaluation measures the student's performance against a predetermined standard. The student is measured without regard to the performance of the rest of the group.

2. Validity means that an instrument actually measures what we intend it to measure. There are different kinds of evidence for validity, including content validity, which can be improved by using a table of exam specifications, and face validity, meaning that an expert review of the questions results in agreement that the questions measure the objectives as intended.

3. A cut score is a predetermined level of minimum acceptable performance.

4. Quantitative assessment is unable to capture nuances of complex human performance, such as affect. However, these items are still of critical importance. Qualitative assessment uses descriptive narratives to portray performance.

5. Mean = 43; median = 43.5; mode = 45; range = 15.

6. Because norm-referenced measurement relies on the performance of a group rather than a standard of performance, unusually high performers may result in competent individuals not being able to pass. Conversely, a group of unusually low performers in a class may make it possible for a student to pass without having attained competence.

Chapter 14

1. Essays are best suited to testing the ability to analyze, evaluate, and synthesize information.

2. The method of evaluation is how information is obtained, such as by observing students or analyzing their work products. The evaluation instrument is used to

guide collection of specific observations and to serve as documentation of the observations.

3. Using corrected true/false items calls for students to rewrite false items to be true, or to explain why they are false.

4. The horns/halo effect occurs when a specific impression of an individual influences the global impression of the individual. Instructors must take care that they are evaluating a student's current, actual performance and not basing evaluations on past impressions.

5. Fundamental attribution error occurs when an individual's behavior is incorrectly attributed to intrapersonal, rather than contextual or situational factors.

6. When class performance on an exam is poor overall, the instructor must consider the effectiveness of instruction, as well as the validity of the exam for the purpose it was used. The instructor must make time to cover information that was not covered adequately and to correct and clarify information where necessary.

Chapter 15

1. Considerations include the depth and breadth of content, accuracy of content, writing style, physical characteristics, reading level, pedagogical features, and technical design.

2. Considerations include perceived versus actual need, currency in terms of state of the industry, amount needed for the number of students, quality, cost, maintenance, realism, and versatility.

3. The use of videos is beneficial when the video is up-to-date and accurate, and consistency and flow of information is critical, such as in skills demonstration. Video can be used to show otherwise inaccessible experiences such as autopsies, and can be used if suitable for the content scheduled when an instructor cancels at the last minute.

4. Some considerations include using a dark background with light text for slides, using serif fonts, keeping the text to approximately 5 or fewer lines, keeping ideas intact, use of main points only, not a duplicate of the text, and purposeful use of graphics.

5. Many students have come to expect an exact handout of the slides used in lectures. This is not a good idea in primary education. It is more helpful to provide a skeletal outline to structure note-taking.

Chapter 16

1. Lesson plans serve to guide and organize the class session, keep the session on track, provide an outline of the content, detail teaching-learning objectives, and provide a basis for evaluation.

2. Lesson plans include a title, description of the audience, date, the name of the instructor, equipment, supplies, and handouts needed, references, timing, objectives, content, activities, and questions.

3. To create a lesson plan it is essential to begin with the lesson objectives and to analyze the audience in order to guide the breadth and depth of content and select appropriate teaching-learning activities.

4. The process for creating a lesson plan begins with objectives. Research based on the objectives provides a quantity of ideas that are later narrowed down on the basis of quality. The information is prioritized and sequenced, and appropriate activities are selected.

Chapter 17

1. The effectiveness of lectures can be improved by using the volume, tone, and rate of speech and pauses to focus learners' attention; taking time to organize the lecture according to the principles of learning using examples relevant to the learners' experiences; helping students organize notes by using a skeleton outline of the main points as a handout; letting students know you will be calling on them to summarize information at the end of the session; following principles of effective communication; and providing a visual frame of reference.

2. Discussion is structured, yet allows student participation. It also allows the instructor to evaluate student knowledge and helps students develop problem-solving skills.

3. Student assignments help increase students' self-directed learning skills.

4. Case-based teaching and learning activities should provide a sufficient contextual framework but should also strategically omit information that students need to learn to seek out.

5. The most appropriate use of games in the classroom is for review and reinforcement.

6. Effective CBI is interactive, provides feedback, and suggests a pace or schedule for the student to follow.

7. Barriers to good communication include preconceived notions, emotions, thinking speed, assumptions, and language (on the parts of both the sender and receiver).

8. Anxiety can be beneficial in energizing your performance, but in excess detracts from it. To reduce anxiety, make sure you are thoroughly prepared, arrive early, keep a noncaffeinated drink nearby, and use physical movement.

9. Facilitation allows students to participate and interact, express their views, fosters their respect for others' views, improves verbal communication skills, and allows student ownership of the knowledge discovered.

Chapter 18

1. Although respect for individual rights is always a concern, a student who is disrupting the learning environment is violating the rights of the group. As an instructor, you have an obligation to intervene on behalf of the group.

2. Physical characteristics of an effective learning environment include seating arrangements conducive to the activities of the class, comfortable temperature, adequate lighting, freedom from distractions, neatness and organization, and adequate supplies and equipment.

3. Emotional considerations in the learning environment include fostering security and freedom from fear of ridicule and harsh criticism, avoidance of unnecessary stress, and provision of challenging but not overwhelming work.

4. All behavior is motivated, and all motivation is internal. Behavior is motivated when it meets an unmet need of the individual. Extrinsic rewards are not motivating unless they have intrinsic value to the individual.

5. Expectancy theory is based on the idea that individuals put forth effort when they expect that their efforts will result in performance and that the performance is related to important outcomes for the individual.

6. Classroom justice theory is based on equity theory, in which individuals are concerned with the fairness of the relationships between performance and outcomes between individuals.

7. The first step in managing a complaining student is to see whether or not the complaint has merit. In any case, the student should be informed if the condition is something that cannot be changed (such as class meeting times or days). If there is merit to the complaint, the student may have a suggestion for addressing the issue. If there is no merit to the complaint often, the student just wants to be heard. Excuses made by students need to be evaluated on an individual basis to establish the credibility of the excuse. It is not fair to punish adults who have legitimate life issues because some students do offer illegitimate excuses.

Chapter 19

1. Effective clinical education takes place under competent supervision and is participative, with minimal time restricted to observation only. The preceptor must apply principles of effective education in his or her interactions with students to ensure reflection on experiences.

2. Purposes of clinical education include the development of proficiency, work-organization skills, and decision-making and problem-solving abilities; observing role models; developing independence; taking responsibility; becoming socialized into the occupation; and gaining work experience.

3. Characteristics of effective preceptors include: effective communication, interest in students, enthusiasm, organization, teaching skills, clinical competence, ability to provide feedback, open-mindedness, and respect for others.

4. Laboratory learning is best transferred to clinical practice when in takes place under authentic conditions.

5. Lab scenarios must provide adequate contextual information to provide a framework but must not give away information that students need to seek. Lab scenarios must be realistic and pose questions for group discussion.

6. Characteristics of effective lab instructors include skill proficiency, certification at the level of course being taught or higher, positive role models, motivated by teaching, effective in demonstrating skills and giving feedback, and reputable in their EMS service area.

Chapter 20

1. Responsibilities of the program director include: administration of the educational program, continuous quality improvement, long-range planning and continued development of the program, cooperative involvement with the program medical director, and delegation of responsibilities.

2. Responsibilities of the program medical director include: reviewing and approving educational content for appropriateness and accuracy, reviewing and approving the quality of medical instruction and student evaluation, reviewing and approving the progress of each student throughout the program, attesting to the competence of all graduates in all domains of learning, cooperative involvement with the program director, and delegation of responsibilities as appropriate.

3. Faculty are responsible for coordination and delivery of instruction and assessment of student achievement. There may be other responsibilities, depending upon the type of institution in which faculty are employed.

4. Relationships with administrative support personnel can be facilitated by the following: say please and thank you, ask rather than demanding or order, allow autonomy, give sufficient lead time for tasks, consider his or her overall workload, avoid asking him or her to do things you really should be doing yourself, and show appreciation.

Chapter 21

1. A résumé is used when applying for most jobs outside academia. It is a brief, one-page document that emphasizes the highlights of one's career and education. A CV is generally required for academic positions and is a detailed document that describes education, work experience, publication, research, and other professional activities.

2. Prepare for the interview by researching the organization, evaluating your strengths, and anticipating questions that may be asked and how you will answer them. Men and women should both dress in business attire (suits). Make notes about the questions you have and strengths you want to emphasize. Take the opportunity to observe the culture of the organization.

3. Professional development can be both formal and informal. Some good ways of continuing professional development include attending conferences and workshops, reading professional literature, writing for publication, or pursuing formal education.

4. There are many benefits to belonging to professional organizations. These include receiving information via publications and listservs, professional development opportunities, and networking.

Index

National Highway Traffic Safety
 Administration (NHTSA), 6, 9
National Registry of EMTs (NREMT),
 48, 133
National Safety Council (NSC), 49, 133
Needs:
 analysis, 127–28, 146
 hierarchy of, 91–92, 279–80
 learning and, 83–84
Neonatal Resuscitation Program
 (NRP), 49
Networking, 311
Neurolinguistic programming, 85, 87
Normal distribution, 198, 201
Norm-referenced measurement, 191–92

Objectives:
 behavioral, 154
 differences between goals and
  competencies and, 152–54
 enabling, 9, 153
 evaluation and, 159–61
 lesson planning and teaching-
  learning activities and, 157–59
 terminal performance objectives,
  120, 122, 153
 using competencies to write, 154–57
Occupational analysis, 132–33
Occupational Safety and Health
 Administration (OSHA), 35

Patient information, access to, 33
Patient injuries, 31–32
Pedagogical features, 241
Pediatric Advanced Life Support
 (PALS), 44, 48, 49
Pediatric Emergencies for Prehospital
 Providers (PEPP), 49
Pediatric Prehospital Care (PPC), 49
Performance:
 assessment instruments, 222–30
 evaluation of, 220–30
 gap, 146
 measuring, 191
Personality, learning and, 89
Philosophies of education:
 behaviorism, 21
 humanism, 20–21
 progressive, 17–20
Philosophy:
 defined, 17
 purpose of, 14
 versus theory, 15–17
Phonological loop, 103
Physiological needs, 91
Piaget, Jean, 79
Plagiarism, 33–34
Polanyi, Michael, 293
Portfolios, 230, 232, 313
Postconventional morality, 40

Postformal stage, 80
PowerPoint® presentations, 245–47
Practice analysis, 132–33
Preceptors, 290–91
Preconventional morality, 40
Preferences (learning styles), 68–69,
 85–89
Prehospital Trauma Life Support
 (PHTLS), 44, 48, 49
Prescriptive curriculum, 123
Preservice education courses, 47
Primary education courses, 47
Primary instructors:
 defined, 55, 61–62
 roles and responsibilities of, 62–64
Problem-centered learning, 84
Procedural justice, 280, 281
Professional development, continuing,
 311
Professional journals, 60, 313, 316
Professional organizations, 311–12
Proficiency, 289
Program, use of term, 56
Program evaluation. See Evaluation,
 course/program
Progressivism, 17–20, 105–8
Proxy, 159
Psychomotor, 10, 11
Psychomotor domain, 111, 114, 293–95
Psychosocial development, 77–78
Publication, research and writing for, 318
Public domain works, 34
Public speaking, anxiety and, 271–72

Qualitative assessments, 186, 195
Quantitative assessments, 186, 195
Questionnaires, 185–86

Range, 198, 200
Rating scales, 226–29
Reading level, of textbooks, 240–41
Realistic job preview, 317
Receiver, 269
Recertification, 48
Records:
 access to educational, 33
 maintaining, 65–66
Reflection, 108
Refresher education, 47, 48
Reliability, measurement, 192–95
Remediation, 233–35
Respect, 59
Responsibilities:
 defined, 62
 of primary instructors, 62–64
 of secondary instructors, 64–66
Rest, J., 39
Restricted-response essays, 209, 210,
 211
Résumés, 313, 314

Risk management, 35–36
Roles:
 defined, 62
 of primary instructors, 62–64
 of secondary instructors, 64–66
Romiszowski, Alexander, 294

Safety needs, 91
Scheduling, clinical, 291–92
Schema (schemata), 14, 103–4
Secondary education, 45
Secondary instructors:
 defined, 55, 61
 roles and responsibilities of,
  64–66
Selection items, 209
Self-actualization, 92
Self-confidence, 58
Self-directing, 82–83
Self-esteem, 92
Self-evaluation, 72–73
Self-motivation, 57
Semantics, 269
Semesters, 164–67
Sender, 268–69
Sensory memory, 102–3
Sexual harassment, 29–30
Short-answer items, 209, 210, 211,
 217–18
Short-term memory, 103
Similar-to-me effect, 232
Simpson, E., 294
Skill development, stages of, 294
Skills checklists, 224–26
Social learning, 16
Social needs, 91–92
Social perception, 232
Specialty certification courses, 48–49
Stakeholders, 122
Standard deviations, 192, 193
Standard of instruction, 29
Stereotypes, 232
Students:
 advocacy, 61
 assignments as a method of learning,
  265–67
 complaining/excuse-making, 284
 conduct/discipline issues, 34–35,
  278–85
 dependent, 284
 evaluation of, 207–35
 grades, expectations of, 204
 grades, posting of, 33
 hostile/confrontational, 282
 injuries, 30–31
 measuring performance of, 191
 motivation, 278
 nonparticipating, 284–85
 performance, evaluation of, 220–30
 records, access to, 33